THE FAST WALK

MOVING AWAY FROM FOOD AND
CLOSER TO JESUS THROUGH FASTING

Louis Trinca-Pasat

THE FAST WALK
Moving Away from Food and Closer to Jesus Through Fasting
Copyright © 2025 by Louis Trinca-Pasat

Cover Design by Abigael Elliott, Interior Layout by Suzanna Chriscoe

ISBNs: 979-8-89165-229-3 ebook
         979-8-89165-230-9 Paperback
         979-8-89165-231-6 Hardcover

Published by: Streamline Books
Kansas City, MO
streamlinebookspublishing.com

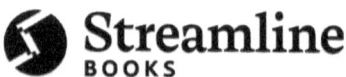

To Jesus.

But I do not account my life of any value nor as precious to myself, if only I may finish my course and the ministry that I received from the Lord Jesus, to testify to the gospel of the grace of God.

—Acts 20:24

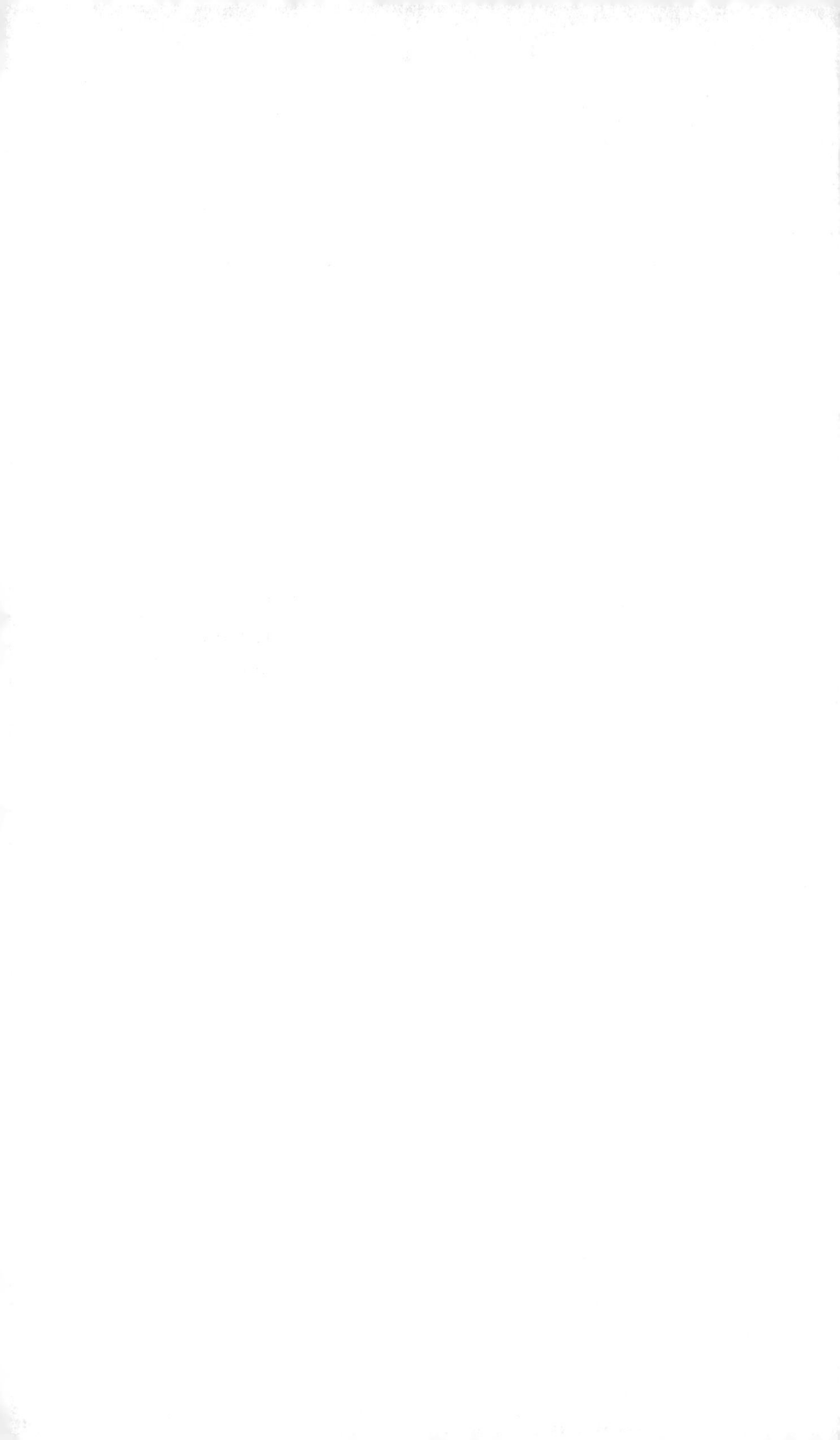

CONTENTS

INTRODUCTION

The steps of a [good and righteous] man are directed and established by the Lord, And He delights in his way [and blesses his path].

—Psalms 37:23 (AB)

The journey that would utterly transform my life began in June 2019, nearly two years after I got cut from the Los Angeles Rams and my professional football career came to an end. Despite no longer being an active player, I was still carrying around the weight of a 295-pound defensive tackle. I had no reason to maintain the weight, and it didn't feel good any longer to be that size. Something had to change.

Around that time, I learned that my brother, Vasile, had adopted a vegan diet. I initially made fun of him for it. It seemed extreme and wholly unnecessary. He insisted that his new diet made him feel healthier than ever. He encouraged me to watch two documentaries, *Forks Over Knives* and *The Game Changers*. These films highlight the benefits of a vegetarian diet for athletes and expose the harsh realities of the meat industry.

Up to that point, meat had been a staple in my diet. Most of my meals consisted of only meat with a few veggies. However, I was intrigued by what I learned from the documentaries. I wasn't ready to permanently embrace a vegan diet, but I decided to try it for ten days and see how I felt. The initial days as a vegan were rough, but by the seventh day, I began to feel a significant improvement in my health. I had more energy, I felt lighter, and I was more comfortable in my body.

Encouraged by this positive change, I decided to stick with the vegan diet, and I incorporated running into my routine. Within three months, I had lost seventy pounds, dropping from 295 to 225. This physical transformation marked the beginning of my *physical* journey toward a healthier lifestyle.

During this same period of time, I was also desperately seeking a purpose in life. My football career was behind me. I was left questioning my identity and the meaning of my life. I really didn't know who I was anymore. Who was I without football? Every night, I would earnestly pray for guidance, pleading with Jesus to reveal His plan for me. Occasionally, I added fasting to my praying in the hopes that I would receive an answer from the Lord, but the longest I ever went without food was three days.

Not long after, I signed up for a mission trip to the Philippines. That trip proved to be a monumental turning point for me. I had a profound encounter with Jesus in the mission field, and He changed me in ways I had not anticipated and never dreamed possible.

On February 8, 2020, there was an altar call at church. I went up front, cried out the name of Jesus, and it was as if time had stopped at that moment. I could have heard a pin drop. At that moment, Jesus revealed Himself to me. I saw a vision of His hand coming from the clouds, His finger pointing directly at my heart. As His finger got closer to my chest, I felt the sin parting from my heart. There was a soft, gentle, caring voice. He said, "Louis, I don't care about what you did. I died for you, and I love you."

In that moment, as I encountered Jesus and felt His love, I thought, *How could God still love me despite all the messed up things I've done in my life?* That's when I told Him, "I'll do anything for you, Jesus." That was the day I finally fully made Jesus my Lord and surrendered my life to Him.

He freed me from the bondage of lust, depression, religion, anger, and an addiction to pornography I'd had since the age of twelve. He gave me a clear directive: "Louis, go preach the gospel and reach the unreached. Go to the hardest places where no one goes."

In the Philippines, God's love moved from being merely a concept in my head to becoming a tangible reality in my heart. I came to realize that His love was not contingent on my actions. He was not chiefly concerned with my outward behavior. Above all, He desired my heart and to have a personal relationship with me.

At the same time, my religious barriers crumbled, and my boxed-in perception of God, shaped by my upbringing in a single church, was shattered. God transformed my heart, revealing its flaws and demonstrating His boundless love for people. I witnessed Him working through different individuals to spread the gospel.

Since surrendering my life to Jesus, I found myself hungry and desiring to know Him on deeper levels, so I pledged to do anything for Him. I returned from the trip with a newfound hunger for Jesus. This marked the beginning of my walk with Jesus, the Only Living God. A quest that began as a search for physical health had become a path to a deeper spiritual life with Jesus.

Fasting for Revival

From that point on, I had no desire for or interest in the worldly distractions that used to captivate me. I sold my video games and removed anything that would distract me from Jesus, and I immersed myself in the Scriptures. I intentionally developed a habit of reading the Bible from cover to cover.

Around that time, I also reconnected with an old friend, Colin Goebel, via social media. Colin was a former teammate of mine from the University of Iowa. I remembered him as a quiet, reserved young man. Now, he appeared utterly transformed on social media: lean, healthy, and with a bold testimony of his newfound faith in Jesus. Seeing the changes in his life ignited my spirit. I reached out to him on Facebook and discovered that he lived in Chicago, where I was residing at the time.

We were right in the middle of the COVID era, but Colin paid me a visit. We shared our testimonies, and he gave me a copy of the book *Atomic Power with God, Thru Fasting and Prayer* by Franklin Hall. Although I appreciated the book, I initially put it on a shelf and forgot about it.

As I continued to let Jesus guide my path, the pastors from the Philippines mission trip suggested I go to seminary. I learned about Dallas Theological Seminary in April of 2020, and the following month, I started classes online before moving to Dallas in August of that year.

I signed up for four classes, twelve credit hours. My hunger for Jesus was insatiable. Eventually, I picked up the book Colin had given me. As I read it, I found myself immersed in the testimonies of individuals who had fasted for fourteen, twenty-one, and up to forty days. Some had even gone as far as fasting for sixty days, consuming nothing but water for the duration of the fast.

But the most amazing part of the book was the stories about revivals in the 1940s. People would gather to worship Jesus in tents, with the heavy presence of the Holy Spirit, and many found healing and deliverance. It didn't matter who they were or what they were grappling with. The evangelist, fueled by his own prayer and fasting, was channeling the power of the Holy Spirit, and it resulted in miraculous healings and people surrendering their lives to Jesus.

These revivals resonated deeply with me. I felt as though I had found the answer I was seeking. I wanted to know Jesus and serve Him in a powerful way, and more than that, I wanted to make Him known to other people. I decided to follow Franklin Hall's advice and commit myself to prayer and fasting.

As I said, the longest I had ever fasted was three days, but when I read about these longer fasts, I realized I was missing out on something far more profound. In fact, it felt a bit like playing a video game and unlocking a secret level. Maybe you know the experience. Your video game character is wandering along a path when you stumble upon a hidden tunnel that leads to an entirely new level, and suddenly, you've unlocked a part of the game that was previously hidden from you. This was how I felt when I realized it was possible to fast for a lot more than three days.

The book also discussed the benefits of weaning off certain foods, particularly meat, and adopting a fruit and vegetable diet before embarking on a long fast. Coincidentally, I was already following a vegan diet. It was as though Jesus had been preparing me for this fasting journey all along, using my choices for His glory and bringing me closer to Him.

With this newfound understanding, I knew what I had to do. On May 25, 2020, I embarked on my first long fast. For twenty-five days, I consumed nothing but water. Because of COVID, I spent most of that time in my parents' basement, seeking the Lord. The first five days were a struggle, but I persevered.

Throughout my fast, I continued taking seminary classes. In fact, surprisingly, the fasting process made me feel more alert and focused for my classwork. I was able to complete two of my courses during the twenty-five days—a testament to the power of fasting and the profound impact it had on my life.

A Guide for Changing Your Life

After that, I read more books by Franklin Hall. His unique perspective on fasting intrigued me, and I found myself devouring his books one after another. As time went by, my hunger for understanding has only grown, leading me to seek out and read every book on fasting I can find, from the secular to the spiritual, from medical to metaphysical.

Despite my extensive reading, I discovered a noticeable gap in the literature on fasting. There is a lack of practical guides that help readers go through a long fast and detail the spiritual, physical, mental, and emotional journey they might experience. This realization sparked a desire within me to fill the void, to create a guidebook that could help anyone and everyone understand what fasting is, how to prepare for it, and what to expect. The book you're reading right now is the fruit of that calling.

I believe fasting is more than merely a form of self-discipline. It's a vital spiritual practice straight out of the life of Jesus that has been overlooked in modern times, and it has become shrouded in misconceptions and misunderstandings. In this book, I hope to clear up these misconceptions and illuminate the true transformative power of fasting.

Embarking on a fasting journey can change your life. I say this from personal experience. A fast of more than twenty-one days alters your perspective on food, deepens your understanding of Jesus, and takes your spiritual growth to a whole new level. If you make it through a forty-day fast, you will no longer be a lukewarm "Christian" but a true follower of Jesus with a profound understanding of the Bible, the spiritual realm, and living a life fully surrendered to the Holy Spirit.

I can tell you all of these things, but true knowledge only comes from experiencing it yourself. When you go through a fast, your faith is built day by day as you wrestle with the flesh. I believe in the importance of personal experience, of living and breathing the teachings I share. In fact, before I began writing this book, I knew I had to embark on a forty-day fast myself. I had to put weight and authority behind my words. So that's exactly what I did.

This Book Is for You

Ultimately, fasting is not about the physical benefits—although it offers many physical benefits (as we will see)—or achieving some personal goal. Rather, at its heart, fasting is about seeking the Lord and growing in the knowledge of Him.

If you've ever felt stagnant in your life, lacking purpose, plan, or identity, if you're clouded and confused, seeking truth, or needing a fresh hunger for God, this book is for you. God is so vast and mighty (Isaiah 40:28; Psalm 145, 147:5) that even eternity will not be enough time to fully comprehend Him (Revelation 1:8, 22:13). Therefore, there must be more to Him that we can discover while we are in our earthly bodies.

Fasting is a means to discover God on new levels and in new ways. It is a practice that aligns things in your life without any effort on your part because your heart's desire is to see God, who draws close to those who draw close to Him (James 4:8).

Food is the third greatest need we have, after air and water, so when you deny yourself food for a set period of time, it is a profound statement of desire to seek and serve the Lord above all else. When you fast, accompanied by prayer and a sincere heart to know the Lord, you will encounter Him in ways you never have before.

I also intend this book for church leaders. Even though fasting was a regular practice of the early Christian community, the vast majority of pastors today have never fasted more than one day or don't see a need for it. And we wonder why there is such a lack of power in churches, why so many churches are fading, and why the next generation is one of the most churchless generations we've had in this nation.

We have churches that are full of teaching and Bible knowledge but lack the power of God and the flow of the Holy Spirit. People come into these churches and leave the same person, even after attending for forty years, still living in bondage to sin and trapped in the same unhealthy patterns.

I believe church leaders are burning out and becoming passionless because they are trying to build God's kingdom in their own strength. Fasting is one significant way that will get you to stop trying in your own strength (pride) and instead allow yourself to be led by the Holy Spirit (humility). Again, I know from my experience and the experiences of many others that fasting leads to healing in the soul, a spiritual renewal of fire and hunger, and a building of faith.

So right up front, I'm putting out the challenge. I encourage you to fast and watch your faith skyrocket. Ask Jesus to give you a burden to fast. Commit to a fast of twenty-one to forty days—a true biblical fast of nothing but water—and you will see your own faith, your confidence in the Lord, and the power of God increase in a powerful way.

In essence, this book is my call for every follower to seek Jesus through fasting, and I'm confident that if you do so, you will find Him. I didn't write this for any specific church or denomination. Fasting is not about the charismatics, the Calvinists, or some particular school of theology. It is a biblical practice that is intended for everyone who is seeking the Lord. It is a call for unity and humble hearts because

God is a God of unity and peace, and He will bring unity to the body of believers if we desire it.

Fasting can unify everyone, regardless of their theological beliefs, and can benefit all religious groups. Since the beginning, people have tried to understand God. They've taken the Bible and interpreted certain Scriptures to come up with an understanding of God. Today, according to the World Christian Database, there are over forty-five thousand denominations worldwide.[1]

I was once guilty of thinking God operated in a specific way. I grew up in a Romanian Pentecostal church, and I thought you needed to speak in tongues to be saved. However, not only is this not true biblically, but I've witnessed people who never spoke in tongues but had the fruit of living for Jesus, even to the point of death. Through my fasting journey, I asked God to teach me His theology. While fasting, God led me to different countries, people, and churches and showed me that He operates in ways my mind can't comprehend. He does what He wants.

There's a mysteriousness about God, but at the center of it all, He wants a personal relationship with every human heart. He wants you to have His heart and mind in all things. Fasting will bring you to a place where you lay aside your understandings about God taught by people and let yourself be taught by Him. It takes you out of the box and puts you into His hands. Even those who do not identify with a particular religion can benefit from fasting, as Jesus Himself was not about religion but relationship.

And, yes, there are physical benefits to fasting. I believe it can lead to healing in the body. In fact, I will be bold enough to say that I believe fasting can help you overcome almost any sickness or disease, but many people turn to fasting too late after trying every other form of medical intervention. We trust more in medicine, which often simply masks disease rather than truly healing them, even as we continue unhealthy eating habits that lead to obesity, sickness, and disease.

Isn't it interesting that the first book of the Bible tells us sin originated from a decision about eating food? God told Adam and Eve not to eat fruit from a specific tree but driven by pride and temptation, they ate it anyway, and it led to the downfall of the world (Genesis 3:6). The decision not to eat for a set period of time is a bold choice to say no to our human appetites, and that can break us from sinful habits or reveal idols we didn't know were consuming our lives.

In my own life, fasting helped me break free from an addiction to pornography that had plagued me since childhood. I started using fasting to deal with the temptation. Every time I felt tempted, I would fast, sometimes up to three days, until the temptation subsided. Over the course of two years, this practice caused the temptation to diminish and eventually led me to complete freedom. It reminds me of Mark 9:29, where Jesus says, "These can only come out by prayer and fasting." If you are struggling with habitual sin or strongholds, these are signs of demonic oppression. When the demonic has become part of your life through sin, generational iniquities, or inner wounds of the heart, sometimes the only way to freedom is by fasting.

This is the kind of power that so many people, including pastors, are missing out on, and it's why so many are living in defeat. If you are struggling with your sin nature or are sin-conscious (trying to do everything you can not to sin), the power of fasting will change your perspective and give you the mind of Christ (1 Corinthians 2:15). You will walk in freedom away from desires to sin because Jesus has given every believer this freedom (Luke 4:16–21; 1 John 3:8; John 8:36). I want to help you discover that power.

There are times when you might find yourself praying for a particular outcome, perhaps for a change in your marriage or overcoming an addiction. You might pray for years, even decades, without seeing any tangible results. Fasting has the power to shatter the chains of bondage and help you break free from the oppressive forces that are holding you captive.

And it's not a practice limited to individuals. Churches, educational institutions, Bible colleges, and seminaries can all benefit from community-wide fasting. Many people aren't taught about it, so they don't understand the purpose or the practice of fasting. They see it as an outdated practice, meant only for the disciples of the past. Others might have a distorted understanding of what fasting truly entails.

We're going to delve into these misconceptions in the first chapter of the book because I want you to understand that *anyone* can embark on a twenty-one- to forty-day fast. And if you do, I believe you will experience a profound transformation. You will never view food or your body in the same way again, and your experience with God will be profound. Each fasting journey you embark on will bring a new revelation of God's character and understanding of the Bible. The power of fasting can make an impact beyond your own experience, even impacting many generations to come.

If you desire such a transformation in your life, then you've come to the right place. Let's go on this journey together and begin a walk that will change your life.

CHAPTER 1: WHAT IS FASTING?

The story of Jonah is inspirational. No, not the part where he gets thrown into the sea and swallowed by the big fish. Actually, it's the story of the people of Nineveh that moves me. Jonah, a minor prophet, is sent by God to Nineveh to prophesy against the city because of the wickedness of its people, but Jonah harbors a deep dislike for the city and wants nothing to do with the assignment.

Nineveh, according to the *Lexham Bible Dictionary*,[2] was the capital of the Assyrian empire during its period of dominance in the ancient Near East, around 703 to 612 BC. Located on the banks of the Tigris River, it was a thriving eastern city under the rule of a powerful conqueror named Sennacherib. In biblical literature, Nineveh is often used as an archetype of evil, and indeed, the city was known for its inventiveness in devising new methods of torture and its disregard for God.

Despite their evil ways, the people of Nineveh had the best of everything. They had the finest horses, chariots, and army. The people of Nineveh were fearless, worry-free, and dominant, destroying everything in their path. Their city was thriving with huge walls, beautiful buildings, and all the pleasures you could think of. The people worshiped other "gods," lived for themselves, and cared about satisfying the lusts of their flesh. They gave into every sensual pleasure they desired. America is a modern-day Nineveh.

Today, we have everything we need. We have the best of everything, one of the strongest militaries, economies, and countries in the world. We have nice cars, houses, more clothes and shoes filling up our closets. People can work without getting out of bed simply by putting a pair of high-tech binoculars on their faces. We have all the food we could ever eat or want. We can even have meals delivered right to our doorsteps at the mere press of a button without having to leave the house. We have quick, easy meals cooked by an air fryer or microwave in minutes. Grocery stores on every corner. Snacks at our fingertips to satisfy immediate cravings. Physically working to earn a meal, or waiting, especially when it comes to eating, is a thing of the past. The younger generations are growing up in a society where their sensual gratifications are immediately satisfied. There are hardly any food shortages, famines, suffering, or waiting.

America is thriving, but people have forgotten about where all of these blessings came from. The consequence is people don't feel the need to rely on God. Worse, people think they've earned or created this life without God's help. Slowly, over time, generations got comfortable and bored and started pursuing idols or giving in to the pleasures of sin. God is left out of the picture, sin starts to run rampant in the nation, and people stop fearing the consequences of sin. Everyone starts doing what "feels" right to them. People have become full of pride and have made themselves "god."

In the story, Jonah initially tries to run away from his calling. He doesn't want to deliver God's warning to the people that he considers his enemies. He gets on a ship and tries to run away from Nineveh. However, the Lord intervenes by sending a storm that leads the men on the ship to throw Jonah overboard. God saves Jonah's life by causing him to be swallowed by a large fish. After being entombed in the fish's belly for three days and three nights, Jonah is finally spat out back on dry land. Once again, the Lord instructs Jonah to go to Nineveh and deliver His message.

So Jonah relents. He goes to Nineveh and delivers a simple message: "In forty days, Nineveh shall be overthrown." He doesn't use theological eloquence. He simply warns the people that they are about to be destroyed by God. Amazingly, the wicked people of Nineveh believe Jonah's message. They don't argue, doubt, or mock him. They don't even hesitate. They believe in God, call for a citywide fast, and put on sackcloth, from the greatest to the least of them.

What's remarkable about this story is that *everyone* fasts—from the oldest human being to the youngest baby, even pregnant women and animals. Even the mighty king responds to the message. He removes his robe, covers himself in sackcloth, and sits in ashes, lamenting the state of his city. He then makes a public proclamation, calling all of his people to prayer and fasting in the hopes that God will show them mercy.

A similar situation occurs in Joel 2:12, 15–16, where the prophet Joel, speaking on behalf of the Lord, calls everyone in the city of Jerusalem and the nation of Israel to fast. King Jehoshaphat also called the nation to fast when Judah was invaded (2 Chronicles 20:1–4).

These biblical stories serve as a powerful reminder of the transformative power of faith and repentance combined with fasting and prayer. Can you imagine the American president doing something like this? Imagine a scenario where a prophet, a divine messenger, declared that the United States would fall in forty days.

Would Americans halt their daily routines and declare a time of fasting and repentance without questioning the prophet's credibility? What if every single person in the country responded positively and began to pray and fast? What would be the outcome? Would America, as we know it today, embrace such a call? Imagine if the president stood at the podium for the State of the Union speech and said, "This nation is headed toward God's judgment. Americans are full of hatred for one another. We live for ourselves, and we look for new ways to do evil. We're running away from the love of God, and judgment is imminent. Therefore, I am asking every man, woman, child, and every living thing in America to pause from work or any activity other than to fast and pray for God to purify our wicked ways, forgive this nation, and show us mercy."

Seems pretty unlikely, doesn't it? But that's exactly what happens in the story of Jonah. The city of Nineveh proclaims a fast, which mandates that no one, either human or animal, can consume any food or water. It is their heartfelt plea to the Lord for mercy, an act of repentance and seeking forgiveness.

This is precisely what we need more than ever in every individual's life, family, church, city, state, country, and the world. We all need to pause and declare a fast because we're on a downward trajectory, and we are not immune from God's judgment.

The people of Nineveh don't question the prophecy, and they're not sure there is any hope for mercy. They declare the fast on the mere hope that *maybe* God will forgive them. The proclamation from the king says, "Who knows? Maybe God will relent and withhold his fierce anger so that we may not perish" (Jonah 3:9).

In other words, they're not trying to manipulate God. They don't feel like God owes them anything. They're simply expressing a desperate hope for forgiveness in the face of what they know is well-deserved punishment. And with no certainty about the outcome, they press on, fueled by faith and hope.

By the end of the story, a beautiful transformation takes place. God observes how the people of Nineveh fast and repent, and their act of devotion moves his heart. He sees their journey during this time of fasting as the people go from a state of worldly and wicked living to a state of holiness, pursuing the Lord and aligning their wills with His.

Ultimately, God relents from the disaster He had planned. He decides against it. The text does not specify the duration of their fast, but it doesn't matter. The crux of the story is that the people, despite living in a city notorious for its wickedness, embarked on a fast to repent. They did so promptly, without any doubt, and God responded in a powerful way. The people not only received forgiveness but also gained a revelation of who God is, and they grew closer to Him. Revival broke out in the city. People turned away from their idolatry and their gluttonous, sensual, and lustful lifestyles.

The question now is, are you willing to repent from a life of sin and turn to Jesus through fasting? Do you want to see this country turn to Jesus? It has to start with you falling on your knees. Please read Jonah's book and his declaration to Nineveh and take it to heart. Spirituality, the universe, Mother Nature, crystals, astrology, and even science can't save you. Jewish laws, Muhammad, Buddha, Joseph Smith, Jehovah's Witnesses, Hebrew Israelites, Hinduism, other gods, the pope, the church, religion, and all your religious acts can't save you.

All have sinned (Romans 3:23). We are headed to hell (Romans 6:23). Jesus loves us and showed it by paying for our sins on the cross (Romans 5:8; John 3:16). There's no other God who can save us (Acts 4:12). Surrender your life to Jesus by faith (Ephesians 2:8–9). Ask Jesus to give you that same sense of urgency, repentance, and humility as the people in Nineveh. Stop living for yourself. Hunger for Jesus and start fasting. Ask Jesus to purify your life. Yes, you can have a relationship with your Creator starting today (Romans 10:9–10).

"If my people who are called by my name humble themselves, and pray and seek my face and turn from their wicked ways, then I will hear from heaven and will forgive their sin and heal their land" (2 Chronicles 7:14).

The Meaning of Fasting: Hebrew and Greek

The story of Jonah is contained in the Old Testament, which was written primarily in Hebrew. In fact, it is from the Jewish people of that time period that we inherit the spiritual concept of fasting. Let's explore the profound meaning and significance of the Hebrew word for "fasting." My research led me to the Hebrew word *tsom*, or *tsum*. This word, at its most basic level, means to abstain from food.[3]

However, an interesting interpretation I encountered suggests that fasting is about covering your mouth to prevent anything from entering—a concept inherently linked to food and the act of self-denial.[4] The root words in Hebrew associated with *tsom* or *tsum* depict an image of an individual lying on his side or searching for water.

This interpretation of the word suggests a posture of prayer and the necessity of humility. In ancient times, most people didn't have advanced water systems where water would flow from a pipe into a cup. They had to stoop down at rivers and lakes, fill their jugs, or drink from their hands. This posture of bending down and moving forward on their knees to drink symbolizes humility and prayer.

Therefore, fasting is not just about refraining from food. It also embodies a posture of humility, prayer, and being grounded. You can't be in motion while trying to drink water. You can't run. You have to be stationary, anchored in a place for a moment, to achieve something. Even though you're anchored in a place and perhaps not moving, there's still something happening.

This concept is also mirrored in the English word "fasten." Take the example of being on a plane. During turbulence, a pilot will instruct the crew and passengers, "Fasten your seat belt." Why? So no one will be ejected from their seats or collide with other objects or people. Flight attendants have to sit down and can't serve food until they're released, so they're confined to a spot when the seat belt sign is on. Once they're released, they're free to move about.

In a similar way, fasting involves being fixed or "fastened" in place until a certain outcome or result has been achieved—until the "turbulence" has passed. Once there's no more turbulence, then you're released. You're free. You can move. So there's this idea of intentionally choosing to adopt a posture of humility and anchoring yourself in a certain place in the sense of not eating—*waiting* until God turns off the "fasten seat belt" sign, releasing you from the fast and allowing you to eat again.

Now, these are ideas we can glean from the Hebrew word for "fasting." The New Testament, however, was written in a language called Koine Greek. What can we glean from the profound meaning of "fasting" in Koine Greek?

The word for fasting in Koine Greek is *nesteuo* in the New Testament. *Nesteia* signifies the act of abstaining from food, specifically for religious or devotional purposes. However, I see it as more of a relational act, a pathway to grow closer to Jesus, much like someone deeply in love. As Christians, we fast for spiritual purposes, so it is a blend of abstaining from food and pursuing spiritual growth. This is not a new idea—it has always been the core of fasting in the Bible.[5]

Beyond the biblical languages, what can we glean from our own language, English? The English word "fast" stems from the Hebrew and Greek root words found in the Bible. Its definition encompasses abstaining from all food: refraining from eating and denying yourself sustenance. However, in today's society, the term "fasting" has been somewhat distorted to mean abstaining from almost anything. People will say they're fasting from TV or social media or they're practicing intermittent fasting or fasting from certain foods. This is not what the term originally signified.[6] Its original meaning was specifically to abstain from all food for a period of time in order to seek God.

According to Arthur Wallis in his book *God's Chosen Fast: A Spiritual and Practical Guide to Fasting*:

When people do not like the plain, literal meaning of something in the Bible, they are tempted to spiritualize it and so rob it of its potency. Once the truth becomes nebulous, it ceases to have any practical application. They have blunted its edge; it can no longer cut. In the main this is what the professing church, and evangelicals in particular, have tended to do with the biblical teaching on fasting.[7]

Interestingly, the word "fast" also refers to the concept of speed. A car goes fast. This is relevant because fasting and speed are interconnected, as fasting can yield quicker results. As mentioned earlier, someone can pray for something for a long time and see no progress. However, engaging in a three-day, fourteen-day, twenty-one-day, or forty-day fast can result in an acceleration of growth and a deeper relationship with Jesus—growth that is more significant than what you might experience in a lifetime of merely attending church and only praying but never fasting.

In your everyday life, you may feel like you're not progressing or much isn't happening, especially in today's fast-paced world, but the act of fasting can make it feel like the world is spinning a million miles an hour around you. In reality, the world isn't moving any faster; rather, you are advancing at warp speed spiritually. The knowledge and revelation you gain of God and His Word and the growth that comes with fasting can be profound. Someone can pray for healing from addiction for years and not overcome it, but with a twenty-one- to forty-day fast, they'll find they suddenly have no more craving for that addiction. I have seen and heard of these kinds of testimonies many times, and yours is waiting to happen.

Misconceptions About Fasting

Chances are, you have some misconceptions about fasting—what it is, what it means, and what it does—that have been instilled in you over the years. I held many of these misconceptions myself at one time, so let's address them.

My introduction to fasting came as a child through my parents. Short-term fasts were a common practice in our church community, observed at the start of each year. These fasts typically lasted from sunrise to sunset—essentially skipping breakfast and lunch, and then breaking the fast with dinner. Time frames like this were taken from biblical examples of Judges 20:26, where Israelites fasted at the beginning of the day until evening.

As a teenager, I participated in these fasts, albeit irregularly. Perhaps once or twice a week, I would observe the sunrise-to-sunset fast. However, the concept of a complete fast, abstaining entirely from food for longer periods and surviving solely on water, was completely foreign to me. It was an idea that had never even occurred to me.

When I grew older and became a football player, any kind of fasting was a rarity for me, especially before games. I was told I needed to eat enough food to have energy and perform well. Looking back, this is ironic because, contrary to popular belief, fasting before games can actually enhance performance. It might sound counterintuitive, but when we eat, our bodies expend energy on digestion, which can detract from focus and mental clarity.

I stumbled upon a story in one of Franklin Hall's books, *Glorified Fasting*, about an undefeated fencer who attributed his success to fasting for seven to ten days before each match. When I first read this, I found it hard to believe, but after I began fasting, it made sense. For athletes, fasting produces hormonal changes that lead to increased lean muscle and bone mass, improved recovery time, increased adrenaline, and the capacity for more intense training.[8]

Forty days after completing a twenty-four-day fast, my eighth pro-longed fast within a three-year span, I ran my first-ever half-marathon. Seventeen days later, I completed my second half-marathon. I also noticed a significant improvement in my mental clarity and focus, particularly after entering what I like to call "phase two" of a fast (which we will discuss later).

Is Fasting a Death Sentence?

The real culprit of the death sentence is food. Over half of the deaths in America are linked to poor dietary habits. Heart disease, cancer, strokes, diabetes, hypertension, and obesity all stem from diets that are excessive in quantity but lacking in nutrition. These health issues lead to significant medical expenses, lost productivity, disability, and premature death.[9]

Many people mistakenly believe that fasting for more than three days is extremely dangerous. They interpret the headaches, stomach pains, fogginess, sweating, and other symptoms of withdrawal that accompany fasting as signs of harm. In reality, these are signs of detoxification—the body expelling toxins accumulated from years of unhealthy eating.

"One of the main causes of these degenerative diseases is overcon-sumption of sugary, fatty, starchy, and high-protein foods—foods that have been processed, fried, and further devitalized."[10]

What many view as negative symptoms, such as headaches and nausea, are actually the body's signals that it needs to rest and heal. Instead of eating when withdrawal symptoms appear, we should allow the body time to recover. Animals instinctively fast when they are ill, knowing it helps them heal. Yet, one of the biggest misconceptions about fasting is that the body needs more food when feeling unwell. In reality, the opposite is true.

I highly recommend reading *The Complete Guide to Fasting: Heal Your Body Through Intermittent, Alternate-Day, and Extended Fasting* by

Jason Fung, MD, and *Toxic Relief: Restore Health and Energy Through Fasting and Detoxification* by Don Colbert, MD. These books delve into the medical benefits of fasting and dispel many common myths about its dangers and the effects of food and medicine on the body.

Fasting, while primarily a way of drawing near to God, also has both physical and spiritual dimensions. The Bible tells us we are made of body, soul, and spirit. (1 Thessalonians 5:23). "The Bible does not say the body contains a spirit...but that each person is a spirit and is a body."[11] We are one being with an inner and outer dimension.

When I contracted COVID back during the pandemic, I spent a week in the hospital, and during that time, doctors gave me all kinds of medications. I was taking seven to twelve pills a day, and I felt like I was drowning in a sea of pharmaceuticals. After they discharged me, they gave me a bewildering array of medications and a portable oxygen tank as I continued to struggle with the virus. The side effects of all of this medication sent my anxiety through the roof.

Finally, I reached a breaking point. Desperate, I decided I would fast and seek God with my whole heart. If death awaited me, at least I would face it while fervently pursuing Him. And so, for seventeen days, I fasted.

Miraculously, I was completely healed—not only from COVID but also from all the lingering symptoms like sinus problems and loss of taste and smell. While I attribute my recovery to divine intervention, it was my posture of surrender and devotion that mattered most. My focus was entirely on seeking God through fasting and prayer.

To be clear, I have no medical credentials, and fasting is a practice with ancient roots that modern medicine often overlooks. If you're considering an extended fast, consult your doctor, but remember that wisdom often extends beyond the medical field. Jesus should remain the focal point, as He is the ultimate source of healing and hope.

I am convinced that there is no harm in fasting; rather, it serves as a reset mechanism. During fasting, your body heals itself from sickness, irregularities, and damage caused by previous dietary habits, lack of exercise, medications, and their side effects. And when you invite Jesus into your fast, the potential for divine healing becomes real. Whether on day one or day forty, healing comes in the Lord's timing.

If you're unsure about fasting, consider Jesus as an example. Fully God and fully man, He fasted for forty days in the wilderness, drinking only water. If fasting were harmful, wouldn't Jesus have warned against it? Instead, we see in Scripture that Jesus expects His disciples to fast (Matthew 6:16) and leads by example (Matthew 4:2; Luke 4:2).

What Is a Daniel Fast?

Another common misconception about fasting among believers is that a fast can be partial, only abstaining from certain foods. For instance, when people say they're doing a "Daniel fast," they're referring to the story of Daniel abstaining from certain foods (Daniel 1:8, 1:12, 10:3).

God allowed the great nation of Babylon (modern-day Iraq), led by Nebuchadnezzar, to invade Judah (609–598 BC) and overtake Jerusalem. Daniel and his three friends were among the Israelites taken as captives. They were selected to be specially educated and trained to serve in the king's palace (Daniel 1:4). However, Daniel and his friends didn't want to defile themselves by eating the royal foods.

> . First, many of the foods eaten at the Babylonian court (e.g., pork and horseflesh)…would have been unclean according to the law of Moses (cf. Lev 11 and Deut 14), either inherently or because they were not prepared properly; for example, the blood might not have been drained from the meat (cf. Lev 17:13–14).[12]

Following Daniel's example, people will say things like, "I am fasting from meat," or, "I am fasting from chocolate."

In reality, there is no such thing as a "Daniel fast." It could be more accurately referred to as a "Daniel diet" or "Daniel abstinence." True biblical fasting means going completely without food and consuming only water for the purpose of seeking the Lord. The only passage in Daniel specifically identified with fasting is Daniel 9:3, which says, "Then I turned my face to the Lord God, seeking him by prayer and pleas for mercy with fasting and sackcloth and ashes."[13] In this case, the Hebrew word *som* for fasting is specifically used.

However, nowhere else in chapters 1 through 10 of Daniel is the Hebrew word for "fasting" used. Daniel is simply *abstaining* from foods that were considered unclean for Jews, which were animals sacrificed to other gods, but he did not go completely without eating food. Yes, it was a spiritual act, something he did out of a desire to be obedient to the Lord and not defile himself, but it was not the same thing as fasting. The purpose behind it, which many misinterpret, is that Daniel followed God's law by not eating food sacrificed to idols. "Daniel seems to have engaged in a semifast rather than refraining from eating all food for this three-week period."[14] Therefore, it was not a fast but a form of diet or abstinence because some sort of food was taken into his body.

There still is power in abstaining from certain foods. Daniel and his three friends looked healthier. They received knowledge, understanding, wisdom, and the ability to interpret dreams after ten days of eating vegetables and drinking water (Daniel 1:15–17). Daniel also had a spiritual breakthrough and revelation from God after abstaining from certain foods for three weeks (Daniel 10:2–3, 12).

There was power behind his abstaining from certain foods because he was acting in obedience to God. His intentions were pure. Therefore, a Daniel diet can be a stepping stone to prepare your body for fasting. There is still power in abstaining from certain foods if you're doing it to seek God. If you have a complicated medical history or have never fasted before, embarking on a Daniel diet can clear the way for long, consecrated fasts in the future.

The Belly Can't Be God

One of the greatest yet most overlooked idols is the god of the belly. By the "belly," we mean the physical pleasure specifically tied to lusting after food and sex. People unknowingly give demons a foothold through the worship and idolization of food. We see an example of this in Philippians 3:18–19, which is the only place in the Bible where Paul is identified as crying. In the passage, he calls out false teachers and pleasure-seeking people in the church, enemies of the gospel who are leading people astray. And he says of them, "Their god is their belly."

Fasting was very common in early church communities. Today, it has become incredibly rare. The false god runs rampant in the Western church, especially in lands where there is an abundance of food. You'll hear more pastors preach about their favorite food or people looking forward to their lunch after church instead of gathering to fast and pray. Often, leaders and pastors trapped in this sin lead the people straight into the same bondage.

A few Western churches may talk about true biblical fasting, but most water it down and wrongly teach people they can "fast" from anything they choose or feel comfortable with—not necessarily food—a measly 21 days out of 365 days of the year. The rest of the time, people are consumed with food. While this form of abstinence can have spiritual benefits, it is not fasting. God does see the heart, and there is power in someone choosing to deny themselves a certain delicacy or desire to purposely spend time with Him. However, there's another level of fasting that involves going for an extended period without food, which leads to a greater revelation, intimacy with Jesus, and a whole denial of the flesh (physical appetites and mind, will, emotions).

Overindulgence in food is an act of worshiping the god of the belly instead of the Only True God, Jesus. Most people don't think they worship food. Yet throughout the day, thoughts of planning meals occupy their mind. Schedules revolve around mealtimes. Food becomes a source of comfort. The body craves something—people feed the craving. Exhaustion leads to relying on caffeine. Depression leads to ice cream. Boredom leads to mindless snacking. Food becomes a crutch to conceal internal battles. People put their trust in food without realizing it.

"Though we are not bowing down, singing praise songs, or worshiping our bellies, we may be more ensnared than we think. We may be way more emotionally attached and mentally connected to food than we would like to admit, and without question, we need the grace of fasting to both dethrone this idol and to protect us from it taking root in our lives."[15]

In other words, people are trying to find a compromise between living for Jesus and living sensual lifestyles. Another term for these kinds of people is "carnal Christians." These people aren't ashamed of living overindulgent lifestyles of food and materialism. Paul was adamantly against these people. Today, carnal Christians subtly live the same way by choosing to twist fasting to suit their comforts, and in doing so, they have made food or their comforts a god. This god of the belly has dulled any spiritual sense of the Holy Spirit. People have no idea what it means to be led by the Holy Spirit or have any spiritual discernment. People falsely "prophesy," create doctrines, and teach the Bible from carnality because their bellies are full and this god leads them.

And then we wonder why there's no power, no hunger, and no real fire for Jesus. Churches are dying. People don't encounter the power of the Holy Spirit. The belly quenches intimacy with the Holy Spirit (1 Thessalonians 5:19). People put so much emphasis on not sinning to avoid quenching the Holy Spirit, yet one of the greatest tragedies has been taking a biblical practice and making it more comfortable for us. That is not biblical fasting.

Paul talks about the flesh and spirit working against each other (Galatians 5:16). Fasting, prayer, and denying your flesh are part of being a follower of Jesus. The god of your belly wants to make excuses and find ways to compromise. Fasting doesn't allow the belly to decide or become a god. It allows Jesus to be the only God.

Is Fasting a Form of Starvation?

Another common misconception is the idea that if you fast, you are starving yourself. The assumption is that if you stop eating food, even for just a few days, you are depriving your body of nourishment, and therefore, you are damaging or destroying yourself. This implies harm to the body and self-imposed cruelty with no spiritual purpose attached to it.

But fasting is not an attempt to harm yourself. Rather, it is the denial of food for a select period of time for spiritual purposes. When approached with the right attitude, it does no harm to the body. In fact, during a fast, the body actually consumes a lot of the impurities, diseases, and garbage that has been stored in the body (in a process called "ketosis").

"We store food energy as body fat and use this as fuel when food is not available. Muscle, on the other hand, is preserved until body fat becomes so low that the body has no choice but to turn to muscle. This will only happen when the body is at less than 4 percent."[16]

For comparison, I completed a twenty-six-day fast, my fourth fast of over twenty-one days or more within two years. The National Football League Players Association (NFLPA) provided former players with a comprehensive medical exam. I completed a full-body medical exam seventeen days after my twenty-six-day fast. My starting weight was around 260 pounds, and afterward, it remained consistent at 232.4 pounds. My body fat percentage was around 28 to 30 percent before the fast and 21.8 percent after. My daily metabolic rate didn't slow down much, and I was burning 2,150 kilocalories. Over time, my body has become more efficient in using the food I eat to provide energy. The medical center said I was one of the healthiest former NFL players they've ever had. I share all of this to show you my body was getting healthier, stronger, and more optimally functional the more I fasted and stayed on a diet of fruits and vegetables.

God, in His wisdom, designed our bodies in such a way that when we fast, they do not initially consume healthy tissue, which would indeed be harmful. Instead, the body uses the accumulated garbage, fat, and everything that doesn't need to be there.

That is why most people can go many days without food, just water, because they have plenty in their reserves. Famously, a five-hundred-pound man named Angus Barbieri went 382 days without eating any food. He drank water and took one multivitamin every day. His body lived off his fat, of which he had plenty.[17] I've personally heard of people going sixty to eighty days without food. Their bodies had plenty of junk in reserve to draw from.

Now, let me be clear: Fasting from food *does* become dangerous once your hunger returns and your body signals that it's time to replenish the body with healthy, good food. As we will discuss later, during a fast, your hunger ceases at a certain point as your body uses its reserves, but eventually, the hunger comes back. When it does, then you need to eat. If you continue to abstain from food beyond this point—whether out of pride or trying to beat a record—your body *will* start to consume healthy tissue, which is damaging and leads to malnourishment. And at that point, it does indeed become starvation, but it will take more than forty days to ever get to that point.

So, the clear difference is that fasting is a *voluntary* healthy practice for seeking the Lord, while starvation is an *involuntary* act because there's no way to get food—it's harmful, damaging to the body, and lacks a spiritual purpose.

Is Fasting a Form of Dieting?

Another thing I want to be clear about: Fasting should never be undertaken with the intention of losing weight. Angus Barbieri lost 276 pounds over the course of his year-long fast, but that is not why we fast.

When you embark on your first long fast, your mind tends to naturally focus on the physical experience because it's a new journey. You may be seeking the Lord, praying, and embarking on a fast to grow spiritually, but your thoughts wind up being dominated by what your body is going through. However, fasting should never be primarily about the physical experience, and it should never be used as a way to lose weight.

If you want to lose weight, go on a healthy diet. That way, you not only lose weight but also learn sustainable eating habits for keeping it off.

Losing weight is a byproduct of a fast, of course, but it should never be the focus. Yes, you will lose an average of a pound a day, maybe more, and you will feel amazing. You will look better and more toned, and your skin will look younger. You will put healthy weight back on as you properly break the fast. But the power of fasting is in the spiritual pursuit.

Abstinence Is Not Fasting

Abstinence and fasting are not the same thing. The general *Oxford English Dictionary* defines abstinence as "a practice or discipline of resisting self-indulgence; self-restraint." In the church, abstinence is defined as "a penitential practice, consisting in abstaining from the use of certain kinds of food. It is thus commonly distinguished from fasting, which means the refusal of all, or all but a strictly limited quantity of, food, irrespective of its kind."[18]

Simply put, abstinence is a form of restriction from certain comforts and is not tied specifically to food or the restriction of all food.

Today, the church and people in America have taken a biblical term and action and redefined it.

No one likes to deny themselves food. A person might say, "I love Jesus. I want to get closer to God, but I don't want to stop eating! I don't want to give up this steak that I can have every day or this delicious chicken sandwich from Chick-fil-A that I can have every day. I am never going to give up meat or alcohol. Absolutely not. I'm just going to say I'm 'fasting' from salad, cookies, or candy bars." Other people suit fasting to their comforts: They don't give up food, but instead say, "I'm going to fast from TV." Instead they should say, "I'm going to abstain from TV because I'm seeking the Lord." Getting off social media, not having sex, or not doing something thoroughly enjoyed is not fasting but abstaining.

The thought of not eating food at all for multiple days in a row is completely foreign to the church in America and society today because we live in abundance. So we twist the words to suit our comforts. People have created the term "liquid fast," which means only drinking juice, which is again a mere form of abstinence because juice is a type of food in liquid form, and the body receives nutrients. When someone says, "liquid fast," what they're implying is, "I'm abstaining from solid foods."

Taken literally, the term "liquid fast" would mean not drinking any form of liquid. People also use the term "water fast" to mean only drinking water, but "water fast" would technically mean abstaining from all types of water and only eating food. The correct way of saying it would be, "I'm fasting."

Can there still be power in abstinence? Absolutely. There are rare cases where someone *can't* fast for medical reasons. The person's body has greatly deteriorated through many years of overstuffing and poor dieting. Overwhelmed by sickness, if the person goes into a fast, it may cause tremendous shock to the body through the overworking body trying to detoxify. It would be better to start with a change in diet, abstaining from certain foods. In that case, abstaining from something to seek Jesus will not go unnoticed by Him. Spiritual purpose can be a part of abstinence, but with fasting, the denial of food in order to seek Jesus are tied together, and one can't be done without the other.

Is Fasting Dangerous?

For his book *The Science and Fine Art of Fasting*, Dr. Herbert M. Shelton conducted numerous studies on fasting, with the number of cases reaching the thousands.[19] In fact, it is believed that he supervised at least thirty thousand fasts. In all of these studies, no one died from fasting, even with durations ranging from twenty-one days to as long as sixty or eighty days.

"Dr. Garfield Duncan of the University of Pennsylvania School of Medicine fasted more than 1,300 obese patients without a fatality. Dr. Duncan limited the fasting period to 10–14 days with repeat fasts at varying intervals. Professor Yuri Serge Nikolaev, director of the Fasting Treatment Unit of Moscow Psychiatric Institute, has fasted many thousands of mentally ill patients for 25–30 days without fatalities."[20]

"Can you fast? Yes—it's been done by literally millions of people around the world, for thousands of years. Is it unhealthy? No. In fact, it has enormous health benefits. Fasting is effective, simple, flexible, practical, and virtually guaranteed to work."[21]

Despite widespread concerns that fasting might be dangerous or harmful to the body, it is not inherently true. There are some doctors and medical professionals who argue against fasting, claiming it is not suitable for everyone. However, I believe this resistance to fasting may be influenced by the medical industry's vested interest in keeping people on medication. After all, the pharmaceutical industry is a multi trillion-dollar industry. The second reason is advertising by big food companies. We see it frequently on billboards, on television, in newspapers, on social media, and in just about every other kind of media. They have slowly ingrained the idea that fasting is to be feared and avoided at all costs. The repetition of messages about always eating breakfast, snacking all day long, and never missing a meal creates a false narrative suggesting that constant eating is beneficial and backed by science.

Unlike prescription drugs and food, fasting is free. It is simple, devoid of monetary gain and profit considerations. That may make it less appealing to the business-oriented medical industry. This is one of the biggest problems when it comes to people not fasting. Big medical and food companies don't want you to find out about the ancient and powerful benefits of fasting.

Personally, I have only heard of two instances of death associated with fasting. One instance involved a man who, after a forty-day fast, ate a large steak, which caused complications that led to his death. The other instance involved a person who did not eat food *or* drink water for over two weeks to see how long he could last, which is definitely harmful to the body. Going without water for an extended period of time is *never* recommended. The few instances where people did this in the Bible were generally supernatural events (such as Moses being face-to-face with God on Mount Sinai) or did not last beyond three days (Esther's and Jonah's fasts).

Even with these rare deaths, fasting wasn't the cause of death. The result of death was the action of the individual lacking knowledge on breaking the fast or disregarding biblical and medical wisdom to not go longer than three days without food *and* water. Rest assured, fasting is safe. Personally, I have been on eleven different fasting journeys of fourteen to forty days, none of which posed any danger to my mind or body. On the contrary, I felt better each time.

More importantly, I do not believe that God would have included Jesus fasting for forty days in the Bible without a good reason. If fasting were dangerous, God wouldn't expect us to do it. Remember: in the Sermon on the Mount in Matthew 6, the top three things Jesus talks about are prayer, fasting, and giving. These, I believe, are the key things God expects of us in the practice of our faith.

Therefore, I dismiss any fear or rejection of fasting as coming from the enemy. Fasting is from the Lord, and I want you to have peace about it.

Is Fasting Manipulation?

In my early days of fasting, I sometimes fasted with the hope that God would give me exactly the things I asked of Him. I had a specific selfish motive, and I thought that fasting would sort of twist God's arm to give me what I wanted. The prophet Isaiah talked about the religious people fasting with wrong motives. In other words, it was a religious outward exercise motivated by self-centered desires (Isaiah 58:3–5). In addition, if you fast to show off holiness, get applause from people, or for religious duty, then congratulations: That's the only reward you'll get (Matthew 6:16).

Fasting should never be used to manipulate God into granting you something you want selfishly. God doesn't owe anyone anything. He doesn't have to do anything for you, no matter the amount of prayer and fasting. You can go into a fast with selfish motives, but I guarantee you, if you go into a long fast of twenty-one days or more, God is going to humble you.

Instead, the intent behind fasting should be selfless, with a focus on God's will, not your own (Isaiah 58:6–14). Your goal should be to grow closer to God, to be set free to serve Him and know Him better. All of the things you initially wanted will have no more grip on you. Greed, lust, pride—those things will break, and you'll just want more of Him. You will become content, at peace, and satisfied with God alone.

A Gift from God

I like this quote from Jack Hayford: The Bible does not suggest that fasting is to be thought a means of earning God's favor or of improving one's status with God. Therefore, we do not fast as a religious or a superstitious exercise hoping to gain God's special attention or tip invisible scales of blessing in our direction. We believe every good thing that comes from God is a gift (James 1: 17) and is the product of His grace, not of human endeavor (Ephesians 2:8, 9).[22]

Everything that God gives is born out of His love and His posture of love, not because we have earned or deserved it. Even if you were to fast for eighty days, you still couldn't earn more of God's love. The exact opposite is true as well. Even if you never go on to fast for more than a day or never complete a forty-day fast, God doesn't love you any less.

The right attitude is to understand that God loves you, He died for you, and through Jesus, He paid for your sins (John 3:16). Therefore, you are forgiven by God's grace through faith and not works or striving (Ephesians 2:8–9). The chance to have a relationship with Jesus is a gift through unconditional love. In return, you should desire to give your heart to Him out of love for what He has already done. The reason you can fast is because it's another gift He's given that allows you to draw closer to Him.

The response should be, "I love Him so much that I want to return His love back to Him," rather than demanding, "God, you owe me. Give me this." As a result of this gift, you're going to encounter Him. He is going to bring you to a point where you no longer care about selfish things or the things of the world. Humility and gratitude will fill your heart, and then you're going to start experiencing His closeness, His blissfulness, His beauty.

CHAPTER 2: WHO SHOULD FAST?

"Fasting is a powerful spiritual discipline that has been practiced for thousands of years by various religions and cultures around the world. In Christianity, fasting has been used as a means of seeking God, growing in faith, and overcoming spiritual obstacles."[23]

My first long fast lasted twenty-five days. Around the eighteenth day, I emerged from my room in my parents' basement, where I had been fasting in solitude. My parents, concerned about my well-being, asked me what was going on. I explained to them that I was fasting, which did not sit well with my dad. He cared for me, and with good intentions, he expressed his disapproval and concern for my health.

Despite his own religious beliefs and past experiences with fasting, my dad couldn't understand why I would choose to abstain from food completely. Fast-forward again to the end of 2021. Out of the blue, I received a text from my dad asking me to pray for him. When I called him to find out what was going on, he revealed that he was on day thirty-eight of his first-ever prolonged consecrated fast. He hadn't eaten anything, and he was still working his full-time job as a building maintenance worker.

I was completely taken aback. My dad, who was in his mid-sixties and had initially disapproved of my fasting, had embarked on a prolonged fast of his own. He explained that he had felt compelled to start fasting and had kept it a secret from everyone. According to my mom, the fast had a profound effect on him. He became gentler and calmer, and he started doing more things for her.

But the most profound change for me, being twenty-seven years old at the time, was hearing my father say "I love you" for possibly the first time in my life. My dad came from a tough Romanian communist background, and he had never been one to express his emotions. To be clear, he was a great father who provided for his family and worked tirelessly, but he just wasn't expressive of his feelings. The fast changed all of that.

My dad's fasting story is one of the many, many stories I've heard of people experiencing profound, life-changing transformation as the result of a fast. People can pray for something for decades and see no progress, but the power of a single twenty-one- to forty-day fast can bring about a sudden breakthrough. If my dad had never fasted, I don't know if I would have ever seen him become more open and vulnerable. The fast softened his heart in a way that nothing else ever had.

This transformation may not seem like a spiritual revelation. He didn't see visions or have any prophetic dreams. Instead, the fast brought about a simple working of the heart, which, in my eyes, still holds a tremendous amount of power. The fact that he's now more open, listens, and talks about his emotions is a testament to the miraculous power of fasting.

My brother, Vasile Jr., is another example. He completed his first long fast, twenty-eight days, and I know the Lord worked in his marriage during that time. The fast rekindled the love between him and his wife and strengthened their bond. These are people who, like me, grew up in church and knew Jesus from a young age. Yet, they had never learned about the power of fasting to bring about transformation. Here is his testimony:

I joined Louis and his group to do a forty-day fast. Before this, my fasting experience consisted of several shorter fasts, the longest being ten days. Louis helped open my eyes to the world of a long fast. I realized how vital a protracted fast can be to one's spiritual growth and transformation. I desired to draw nearer to the Lord through this type of fast.

My fast lasted twenty-eight days. Working full time and being active at work and home with three children, my hunger returned before the forty-day goal. Doing a prolonged fast to draw nearer to the Lord and let Him work in my heart has changed my life. Through the suffering and difficulties I faced during the fast, the Lord made me realize that, while I was saved, I'd never truly made Him the Lord of my life.

It was the hardest thing I've had to do so far. However, it has been the most rewarding as well. Even though my wife didn't fully agree with me about doing the fast, our marriage has never been stronger. I realized I hadn't loved her as Christ loved the church; I wasn't the spiritual leader I should've been for our family, and I wasn't living fully for the Lord. All those things were brought to light and addressed because of the fast. I highly recommend and encourage everyone to fast for the Lord.

Fasting reveals things we haven't seen and causes self-reflection. If someone has been blinded to their own sin and pride, fasting can cause them to see it. It enables people to perceive the changes they need to make in their lives, in their relationships, in their habits and choices. Fasting is truly transformational. And for that reason, I believe fasting is for everyone.

Pursuing More of God

Sometimes, even within the church, followers of Jesus can become too comfortable. They grow content with their lives, not necessarily straying from God, but simply stuck in a routine. They go to church, return home, go to work, return home, take care of their family, and repeat. They forget that there's more to seek in God, and fasting is a key to this pursuit.

Fasting is a clear practice in the Bible for spiritual growth and desiring more of God. However, so many followers of Jesus today feel complacent because they have what they need, and they're comfortable. This was my mindset when I was playing football. I had what I needed, I went to God when I needed something, and I was comfortable. I assumed I was saved and knew where I was going. I didn't feel the need to do anything else. But this is how a carnal Christian thinks. The four major appetites before fasting are hunger, sex, greed, and spirituality, with spirituality being the least important—and often almost nonexistent.

A content person doesn't necessarily see a reason to fast. If they reach a point of desperation in their lives, they might consider it, but even then, it will probably be something quite limited—not a true biblical fast.

Very rarely do people these days, even some rather devout followers of Jesus, consider undertaking a true biblical fast. There's a fear ingrained in us by the medical industry and our general culture. We're told we need to eat three meals a day, have our snacks in between, and constantly fuel our bodies. I believe this is actually detrimental to our health. We need to fast more to let our bodies rest, absorb nutrients more efficiently, and do an internal cleanse.

Fasting isn't exciting or flashy. It's not a quick-fix solution. It's uncomfortable. But then again, if working out was comfortable, everyone would do it, and gyms would be filled to capacity with people who look like Hercules. Fasting, on a spiritual level, is warfare. It's challenging, not easy, not fun, and not always exciting. It's difficult having to see and confront your brokenness or changes you need to make in your own behavior. It's a burden, a battle on the front lines. And people often want the results without the battle.

When we have trouble, we are told to pray about things, go to church, ask Jesus, talk to someone about our problems, or listen to a sermon. But rarely are we told, "Hey, you need to win this battle in your life, so go fast for forty days." If you tell most people that, they're likely to think you're crazy.

This was the initial mindset my friend Soleil had until she embarked on the journey of a prolonged biblical fast. Here is her testimony:

> Before my thirty-seven-day fast, I had only fasted one week. I felt inadequate and unprepared to attempt forty days, but the Holy Spirit made it clear that He was drawing me into it. So, after asking Louis many questions about what to expect, I started. Dizziness, nausea, and fatigue were the hardest physical symptoms to cope with. But resisting the urge to fulfill myself with online shopping and Netflix was much more difficult. However, after fighting the temptation for three weeks, my desire for worldly comfort and pleasure was almost completely eradicated. By week four, all I wanted was God's presence. Despite asking for this—more

intimacy with His presence—and praying through a list of a hundred prayers, I noticed no spiritual change during my fast. After breaking the fast, however, I entered the most spiritually grueling twelve months of my life.

During that time, I lost my job, my scholarship, and my housing. I spent time homeless and faced months of lack. I was spiritually abused, slandered, and criticized by my closest friends. Six months into the year, the worst year of my life, God told me why. He revealed that in my fast, just as in life, I had striven for His presence. In my spiritual orphanhood, I saw the fast as a way to earn proximity to God along with all my ambitions and desires. Instead of giving me what I asked for, God allowed everything to be taken away.

And there, in a place of complete brokenness, He showed me that I already had all I needed. What I learned is that in fasting, you will not earn anything you don't already have access to. But He will show you how much you already have, and how near He already is. He knows what you need more than you do. Trust that what happens postfast is purposeful. He is working. When it gets hard, hold on; He has not left you. This seemingly chaotic mess is the very fruit of your fast.

You don't usually hear these kinds of testimonies from fasting. Usually, you hear about how Jesus answered a prayer someone had been praying for ten or twenty years, how He healed them from sickness or fixed their marriage, and so on. In fact, you may wonder how Soleil's testimony is a fruit of a fast. How is losing everything and going through a chaotic mess a good thing? You may even think, *I don't want to fast only to go through trials and lose everything.*

But there is the beauty many people may miss in Soleil's testimony. Like her, you may discover that Jesus has been near to you the whole time, and all the striving, religion, materialism, family, friends, and things of life have been blocking you from encountering intimacy with Him. In His love, He often takes away the distractions, the striving, the self-righteousness through religion, and the things of the world to open your eyes to see His love. In the process of "losing everything," you gain everything from the fast through the revelation that the only thing of real value you need is salvation by faith through Jesus Christ alone. In this, you gain your value from Jesus's love, and you receive a purpose to live fully for Him and a peace that surpasses all understanding.

But fasting is not only for believers. It can be for people who are on the journey of seeking the truth. Maybe they haven't found it yet, but fasting can help open their eyes. However, any person can receive the physical benefits of fasting, but children of God, those who follow Jesus and have a relationship with Him, are the only ones who receive the spiritual gifts and blessings.

The Bible encourages everyone to search diligently for truth. Jesus Himself emphasizes this in John 8:32 when He says, "The truth will set you free." In John 14:6, He then describes Himself as "the way, the truth, and the life" and reveals that the only path to the Father is through Him.

For anyone seeking meaning in life or questioning the existence of God, I believe that a twenty-one- to forty-day fast can lead to encountering Jesus. Whether you already know Him or not, approaching the fast with a posture of seeking God—asking, "Jesus, can you reveal yourself to me? I want to know you!"—can open the door to experiencing God in a powerful way.

Before His crucifixion, Jesus spent time with His disciples on earth. Aware of His impending sacrifice, resurrection, and ascension into heaven, He prepared them for the future. In Mark 2:19–20, Jesus explains that, during a wedding feast, guests don't fast while the groom is present. Celebration and excitement abound. Similarly, when Jesus was physically with His disciples, they celebrated and learned from Him, but they did not fast like the Pharisees. However, once He ascended, He expected them—and all future believers—to fast. As He says in that passage, "The days will come when the bridegroom is taken away from them, and then they will fast in that day."[24]

Fasting Is for You, Now

If Jesus expects you to fast, then you should consider integrating this practice into your life. You don't have to wait for a special sign. Many people say they want to be led by the Lord or wait for a clear indication. However, the Bible is already clear on this matter. Jesus essentially gives you the green light when He says, "And when you fast" (Matthew 6:16). This implies that He expects you to do it.

Some people will point out that Scripture says the Holy Spirit *led* Jesus into the wilderness, and therefore, you should wait until the Holy Spirit leads you to fast. The problem with this approach is that the voice of the Holy Spirit can be silenced by your struggles in the flesh. It goes against your natural inclinations to deny yourself food in order to seek the Lord. Your flesh is never going to agree with fasting willingly. Your body will never say, "Hey, not eating for forty days sounds like the best idea ever. Yes, do it." Instead, your body will resist fiercely, demanding that you fulfill every craving, whether it's hunger, sex, greed, or carnal desire.

The body will always insist it needs food to live, and there will always be that internal struggle. If you wait for a perfect, magical moment or a special spiritual prompting to fast, you might never start. At some point, you need to make the decision to try fasting and seek the Lord along the way. As we will discuss, you can start slowly and take small steps. Just know that fasting is not an extreme ascetic practice reserved for a special group of elite, superspiritual people. It's for all of us. It's for you. Now.

CHAPTER 3: WHY SHOULD YOU FAST?

Let's consider a list of biblical figures and examine why they did or didn't fast (and the outcomes of their decisions).

Jesus Fasted

When you think about the reason for fasting, the most powerful biblical example comes from Jesus. The name Jesus should be enough reason to fast. God Himself, came, subjected Himself to becoming a human, and put His mind, will, emotions, and physical body through a battle so He could empathize with humanity. Before embarking on His public ministry of preaching and performing miracles, Jesus went on a forty-day wilderness journey where He fasted and *was* tempted by the Devil (Matthew 4:1–11; Mark 1:12–13; Luke 4:1–4). For forty days, Jesus was being tempted. Every day in the fast in the wilderness, the Devil tempted Him. While in the desert, devoid of distractions and conveniences, Jesus had only two choices: sleep or talk to the Father. So that's what He did.

During this period, Jesus likely memorized Scriptures, prayed, and deepened His communion with God, learning to hear His Father's voice even more clearly. This is where He learned to have all His needs met by God. The Father's love was enough to sustain and satisfy Him on this earth. After this intense time of fasting and prayer, confronting the Devil, and rejecting his temptations, His ministry began. He returned and began preaching, "Repent, for the kingdom of God is at hand." Jesus was solid in where He got His value of love. He then operated out of love He received from the Father in the fast. Jesus didn't find His identity in the ministry, food, self-seeking pleasure, kingdoms of earth, popularity, or anything of the world. All He needed was the Father.

In John 4, when Jesus meets the woman at the well, He is thirsty after walking many miles in the heat and asks her for a drink of water. While His disciples go to town to get food, Jesus engages in a life-changing conversation with the woman. By the end of it, she runs back to town to tell others about Him. Notice that she leaves her water jar behind (John 4:28), likely because she had tasted the living water Jesus spoke of (John 4:10). Her physical thirst was satisfied spiritually.

Interestingly, when the disciples return with food, Jesus is no longer hungry or thirsty. They wonder if someone brought Him food (John 4:31–33), but Jesus explains that He was nourished by doing the will of the Father (John 4:34). This shows that there is spiritual sustenance in obeying God. Salvation is the living water that flows from within, and when you remain obedient to God's will, this living water will be enough to sustain you (John 6:27).

This example serves as a model for us. So if you ever feel called by God to do something, the first thing to do is fast. Empty yourself. Remove all distractions from this world and spend time with Jesus in prayer and fasting. Learn to find your identity as a son or daughter in Jesus. Learn to have your need for love be met and satisfied by Jesus and not out of the calling, ministry, or any other reason that would be impure, demonic, or selfish. When you empty yourself and totally satisfy every need with the Father's love, then God will begin to use you for His glory. Your motive will be pure: to live an earthly life fully surrendered to Jesus and to bring Him glory.

In our comfortable lives, we often overlook this essential practice. Our mindset should be filled with gratitude and joy for the salvation God has given us, a salvation that allows us to have a relationship with Him now and guarantees us a place in heaven. This gift is not to be kept to ourselves but shared with others, modeling Jesus's approach with His disciples.

Our faith is not meant to be primarily about debating or converting others or about mastering apologetics and Bible knowledge. It's meant to be about spending time with Jesus through fasting, prayer, and reading the Word. This combination empowers us to walk in the power of the Holy Spirit. And when people witness God's power in our lives, such as through healings, they cannot deny His existence. This simple yet profound truth further emphasizes the importance of fasting, a practice that many have yet to experience beyond a few days in their entire lives. Jesus set the standard, and if He, being God, saw the need to fast, how much more should we?

Those Who Failed to Fast

If Adam and Eve had chosen to fast before eating from the tree that God had forbidden, sin wouldn't have entered the world. The Devil found a way to ruin people, and it was through the lust for food. Then God tried to start all over with Noah, a man who walked with God (Genesis 6:9). However, he fell into the trap of overindulgence of food and got drunk (Genesis 9:20–21). This led to one of his sons, Ham (father of the nation of Canaan), seeing him naked, which led to a curse falling on the nation of Canaan (Genesis 9:22–25).

Esau sold his birthright (leadership over the family and inheritance from the father) over a bowl of soup because he was exhausted

(Genesis 25:29–34). This man knew how to hunt, catch food, and cook meals his dad loved (Genesis 27:3–4). He probably could have made something a lot more delicious than a simple bowl of soup, yet his physical appetite was too great to resist. He didn't have the patience to rest. He wanted to satisfy his immediate lust for food. In so doing, not only did he give up his birthright after he ate (and satisfied his physical appetite), but also, it led him to despise his own life.

God destroyed the wicked cities of Sodom and Gomorrah (Genesis 19:23–25) because of sin. What was the cause of this sin? Pride, an abundance of food, a comfortable life, and not helping people in need (living for themselves). The cities no longer sought God (fasting), and food opened the door to self-indulgent lifestyles, which led to sin and ruin. People lived by every physical desire. They did what felt right to them, and sexual perversion was everywhere.

Consider the destructive fruit that came from those who did not fast but gave in to their lustful cravings for food. Let's compare them to those who fasted.

Others Who Fasted

Before Moses had an intimate conversation with God, he fasted for forty days, and he did this twice consecutively (Exodus 24:18, 34:27–28; Deuteronomy 9:9–18). This is the only account in the Bible where someone went more than three days without food *and* water.[25] Important note: this was a *supernatural* fast; no one should go longer than three days without food *and* water, as this will cause harm and could lead to death.

"In this extrasensuous world he transcends the constraints of time and is released from the demand of his physical being."[26] The power of God's presence is sacred, and humans drawn to His presence respond with fasting.

King David fasted several times because of grief in his life because of the loss of friends or family (2 Samuel 1:11–12, 3:31–36, 12:15–23). Most of the Psalms written by David were the results of prayer and fasting (Psalm 35:13, 69:10, 109:24).

The prophet Elijah fasted for forty days on his journey to Mount Horeb when he was fleeing in fear from Queen Jezebel, but he had a profound, healing encounter with God there in a cave (1 Kings 19). Queen Esther fasted for three days, along with her people, to change the king's mind and prevent their massacre (Esther 4:1–17), and later fasted for two days as an act of remembrance when the Israelites were delivered from persecution (Esther 9:1–32). Anna, an eighty-four-year-old prophetess in the New Testament, fasted and prayed in the temple day and night, awaiting the Messiah's arrival, showing that age or gender is no barrier to fasting (Luke 2:36–37).

The apostle Paul, who wrote two-thirds of the New Testament, fasted during significant times in his life (2 Corinthians 6:4–5, 11:27). After his encounter on the road to Damascus, he went blind and didn't eat for three days (Acts 9) Later, he endured a two-week forced fast following a shipwreck (Acts 27:27–33). These are sacred encounters with God. These are moments of encountering God's holiness and acquiring fear and a deep passion to connect with His creation to fulfill His kingdom on earth. Sacred encounters ignite moments of fasting. It's the human response to desire to connect with Him on a deeper level through fasting.

"In Acts 13:2, the apostles fasted after Jesus ascended to heaven, and they experienced a powerful encounter with the Holy Spirit during their fast—an experience we call Pentecost. Most of the progress in spreading the gospel came from the work of the first-century church, and from key individuals who experienced life-changing visitations from God through prayer and fasting."[27]

Throughout church history, many church leaders fasted, including Martin Luther, John Calvin, John Knox, John Wesley, Jonathan

Edwards, David Brainerd, and Charles Finney. There are also lesser-known people from church history, like Pastor Hsi in China, who fasted. First- and second-century church documents, such as the Didache, highlight the importance of fasting, and early church leaders like Polycarp and Irenaeus, both of who learned directly from the apostles, continued this tradition. Other early church leaders like Clement, Tertullian, and Origen also practiced fasting.[28]

Martin Luther translated the Bible from ancient manuscripts to German. John Calvin was a pillar in developing systematic Christian theology. John Knox impacted the church in Scotland and is known as the founder of the Presbyterian church. John Wesley was a primary figure leading the Great Awakening and revival in England and America. David Brainerd was an American missionary to the Indians.

"When Jonathan Edwards preached his famous sermon 'Sinners in the Hands of an Angry God,' people in the audience said that they felt the ground open up and reveal the depths of hell, causing them to cry out to God for mercy and forgiveness."[29]

Fasting was so vital to the early church that it became a ritual to fast twice a week, typically on Wednesdays and Fridays. It was used to mortify the flesh, humble the soul, and help people abstain from sin and worldly passions. Fasting helped combat heresy, blasphemy, and false philosophies, and it facilitated a deeper connection with God. It also moderated appetites and prevented gluttony, a problem even in ancient times that has only worsened with modern abundance.[30]

Today, fasting has largely died off, but it is needed now more than ever. Many churches in Western culture and throughout America have embraced the idea that we do not need to fast today. This has led to doubt and unbelief. From these doubts and unbelief, man-made doctrines and theologies have been created. There are tons of divisions in the body of Christ. Most churches in America today operate like businesses, and attending church is a task to be checked off a list. People live a kind of "comfortable Christianity" that takes on an appearance of godliness but denies the power of the Holy Spirit. Other churches claim to operate by the power of the Holy Spirit, but behind it all are manipulation and selfish motives.

Fasting purifies us of false doctrines and selfish motives. The result is a desire for unity in the body of Christ. That unity comes from putting Jesus at the center and spreading the gospel to every tribe, tongue, and nation. Thus, revival breaks out because people encounter Jesus through the power of the Holy Spirit. Many examples of the power of fasting have been laid out in the Bible and the testimonies of the early church. If every person in the church today would attempt to walk through a journey of fasting for twenty-one to forty days, and consistently fast as often as the early church did, I believe there would be an explosion of the gospel being spread and people surrendering their lives to Jesus.

An Untapped Power

Historical examples of fasting outside of the church also highlight its importance. In ancient Greece, philosophers like Pythagoras required their disciples to fast for forty days before initiating them into spiritual teachings. Plato, Socrates, and Aristotle also mandated fasting for their students, believing that only through fasting could the mind be purified enough to grasp the profound mysteries of life. These men, even though they did not follow or know Jesus, recognized the transformative power of fasting. Religions like Buddhism, Hinduism, Confucianism, and Islam also practice fasting, and there seems to be a shared belief among world religions that fasting opens the way to spiritual revelation by disconnecting the mind from worldly senses.[31]

Fasting has an untapped power because it involves a true denial of the flesh, even for those who may not be doing it for the right reasons. An example from the Bible is King Saul of Israel, who, when surrounded by the Philistines and preparing for war, sought divine guidance (1 Samuel 28). Desperate for a strategy and not receiving answers from God, Saul turned to mediums and necromancers for help. This desperation reflects a common human tendency to seek control and quick answers when God's timing seems too slow.

King Saul disguised himself and sought out a medium to summon the deceased prophet Samuel. The medium successfully summoned Samuel, and the prophet told Saul that the Philistines would defeat him and take the land. At this point, we are told that Saul had fasted before coming to the medium. This act of fasting, even in a misguided attempt to seek spiritual insight, provides an example of the heightened sensitivity to the spiritual realm that fasting can induce.

Even today, in spiritually charged places in Africa and the Amazon, witch doctors often require people to fast for up to five days before visiting them because they believe fasting opens people up to the spiritual realm. Various religions and spiritual practices incorporate fasting to prepare people for profound experiences.

> In South America, the wild savage has his tribal medicine man or witch doctor. In order to become a medicine man, he has to live for weeks without food, and then chews bark, roots, and plants. He also has to go through a ritual of weird and wild maneuvers before obtaining this high position in the spirit realm. He is supposed to control warfare, crop failures, floods, and nearly everything else, and is also supposed to have great influence in the spirit world. If through fasting, a savage is made almost a god in his tribe, how much more ought Christians to fast to have special favor and power with God.[32]

As in Saul's case, desperation often serves as a catalyst for fasting. When people are facing severe hardships, they sometimes turn to fasting as a way to seek divine intervention. It's in these moments of desperation that the human heart earnestly seeks God, even if that means fasting for an extended period of time to find relief and answers.

The Lord works in mysterious ways to capture our attention, often at the last minute. He desires our whole heart and complete attention. He wants to steer us away from mediums, false gods, and other counterfeit sources so we will come to Him, the true source. We see this in the story of King Saul, who, in his desperation, tried to manipulate an outcome rather than waiting on God.

The key lesson is that it's not about getting the answers you want but about seeking God's will, His answers, and His plans. It's about recognizing your dependence on Him and trusting His timing and plan. Through a consecrated prolonged fast of twenty-one days or more, unbelief shatters, you learn patience, and you rest. Your faith skyrockets. The focus turns from the physical realm to the spiritual realm.

Fasting as Spiritual Warfare

King Saul fasted for the wrong reason. There are even some people who fast with bad intentions or for demonic reasons. The enemy often tries to counterfeit what is good and turn it into something negative. I once heard a story that illustrates this rather vividly.

A pastor on a flight was upgraded to first class, where meals were served. He noticed that the man sitting next to him declined his meal, so the pastor jokingly suggested that he must be fasting. To his shock, the man confirmed that he was fasting. He further explained that he was fasting for forty days as an act of black magic to cause pastors and their wives to get divorced in America. The man was actively opposed to followers of Jesus, and he was attempting to use fasting for a destructive purpose. There are stories of witches in Maine who fast and go to the furthest east point of America before the sun rises to cast spells and welcome demonic spirits into America.

These stories should serve as a wake-up call for every follower of Jesus. If people are fasting for wrong reasons, how much more should the followers of Jesus be fasting to combat such spiritual attacks?

These stories convicted me and really made me see the need to fast more, not out of religious duty but to stand firm in spiritual warfare. It spurred a renewed commitment to fasting in my life. It also made me wonder how we can demonstrate the power, presence, and love of God to the lost world. We can't do it in our own strength. Fortunately, I've learned that when I share the gospel, even when I feel weakest, that is when God moves the most powerfully. It's in these moments when I feel inadequate that I turn to the Lord out of a desire to deny my flesh and allow God's power to be displayed.

And when other people see the power of God working through us, they are drawn to Him. This is why fasting is so important—it leads others to the Lord, sparks revivals, and turns our prayers into action by applying Jesus's teachings.

Fasting isn't just about physical denial; it's a deeply spiritual act. In Matthew 17:21; and Mark 9:29, Jesus explains that some evil spirits and strongholds can only be overcome through prayer and fasting. I believe this applies to many kinds of struggles, such as anger, bitterness, and unforgiveness, which can become spiritual strongholds in our lives if not addressed. The battle is not against the physical, but it's in the spiritual realm (Ephesians 6:12; 2 Corinthians 10:3–5).

Fasting helps us become more sensitive to the spiritual realm, to the Holy Spirit, and to His voice. I've experienced this in my own life. As I mentioned earlier, I was addicted to pornography from the age of twelve until I was twenty-seven. My journey to freedom began when I brought the sin into the light, which started a two-year process that culminated in February 2020. Whenever I felt the urge to give in to temptation, I would fast until the desire subsided. This sometimes took one, two, or three days. If the temptation returned, I would eat a meal and start fasting again. Had I known about extended fasts of twenty-one days or more, I would have undertaken one immediately.

There are countless stories of people being completely freed after a ten-, twenty-one-, or forty-day fast. The process involves subduing the flesh and allowing the Holy Spirit to take over and break the strongholds. For me, my breakthrough came after two years because I did not know about fasting for forty days. People have experienced freedom much quicker through longer fasts. These fasts have the power to break demonic bondages, generational curses, and strongholds, often in a single, dedicated period of a twenty-one- to forty-day fast rather than years of struggle.

The power of fasting for spiritual reasons is undeniable. It not only strengthens our own spiritual walk but also equips us to lead others to freedom and revival. I've seen fasting break the bondages of food addiction, greed, drugs, alcohol, sexual immorality, anger, and pride. It reveals the impurities in our hearts, transforming our lives and setting us free to live according to God's purpose and plan rather than being trapped by our pains and wounds. This, in turn, prevents us from passing on these struggles to our children, breaking vicious generational cycles as we learn to conquer temptation.

Fasting also prepares our hearts for worship, making us more sensitive to God's voice in every aspect of life. It ignites a hunger and burning desire to know and experience God in new and profound ways, with each facet of the journey offering unique revelations. We become more sensitive to the Holy Spirit, and we begin to recognize His voice more clearly, understand the Word better, and gain boldness.

Fasting is not an end in itself but a means to a deeper, more intimate union with God. Early Christians fasted for various reasons, including overcoming the flesh and raising money for the poor. They would fast and use the money they saved from not buying food to help those in need. This act of self-denial and helping others brought them closer to God and filled them with His love, peace, and joy. Material possessions and worldly desires faded in importance, replaced by contentment in God's presence.

Experiencing Breakthroughs

These kinds of breakthroughs typically start to become noticeable two to three weeks into a fast. You'll find your emotions stabilizing, your desires for worldly things diminishing, and a deep contentment taking root. Whether it's the desire for a car, money, a house, or fashionable clothes, none of these will matter. Even the desire for ministry success will pale in comparison to the sweetness of being in God's presence. You will feel a profound serenity, joy, and peace because Jesus is all you need.

Fasting also brings mental clarity, cutting through the clutter of anxiety, overthinking, and lies from the enemy. It shatters fears of rejection, people-pleasing tendencies, and a lack of confidence. As you fast, the opinions of others and worldly concerns fade, replaced by the clear voice of the Father. The mental noise—the thousands of competing megaphones—gradually silences, leaving only the Holy Spirit's voice.

In this clarity, you can discern God's will and plan for your life. Even when the enemy tries to attack with lies or temptations, you can easily deflect them. Your faith becomes a shield, protecting you from the enemy's arrows. When fasting, even witchcraft or curses cannot touch you because of the power fasting holds.

Every fasting journey is different, but healing is a common outcome. Fasting can even create new neural pathways in the brain, triggering parts that may not have been functioning optimally. Studies show that fasting helps regulate brain functions, which can lead to creative ideas and quick, simple solutions to problems.[33] It sharpens your mind, enabling you to solve issues swiftly and effectively.

For those struggling with anxiety or lacking confidence, fasting can be transformative. It shatters the fear of other people and builds up confidence. During a fast, you reach a zone where you are no longer worried about what others think. You can easily approach someone to pray for them, ask about their faith, or engage in a conversation that you would typically shy away from.

This process builds both muscle memory and spiritual muscle memory. The Lord molds new character traits within you, and after the fast, you find yourself more confident and able to engage with others without anxiety. This newfound boldness remains even after the fast is over. You have been through the experience and know you can do it again.

Consider the example of Daniel in the Bible. He gained clarity and gifts through fasting (Daniel 10:3), which allowed him to interpret dreams and become the king's right-hand man. His fasting led to significant revelations and a greater boldness, to the point where he and his friends survived being thrown into a fire.

If all of this doesn't motivate you to fast, then you're missing out on experiencing the power of God—something many people overlook today. I urge you to give fasting a try. Even if you can't manage a week at first, keep attempting it. A fast is never a failure; it's about stepping out, trying, and gradually growing in your faith. With each attempt, you'll go longer, and you'll encounter God in new and deeper ways.

Fasting is a journey of growth and learning. It's about having grace and patience with yourself as you discover how fasting affects your body and spirit. Along the way, ask yourself: What is this journey teaching me? What is the Lord revealing? It all begins with deciding to start. Whether you are healthy, sick, desperate, at peace, or simply curious, I encourage you to begin fasting. Your life will never be the same.

CHAPTER 4: THE EXPERIENCE OF FASTING

So what is the actual experience of fasting like? If you've never done a prolonged consecrated fast of twenty-one to forty days, then it might seem like a mysterious and dangerous process. Let me share my own experience during my first-ever prolonged fast of twenty-five days to allay some of your fears.

By the time I began my first long-term fast, the Lord had already prepared me for it through my change in diet and running. He helped me get to the point where I was ready to begin. I told my friend Colin about the fast, and he shared with me that he had previously done an eighteen-day fast. His guidance was extremely helpful since I was about to embark on this journey and had little idea what to expect.

It encouraged me to know someone personally who had gone through a long fast and come out the other side alive and well, and Colin knew a few other people who had done forty-day fasts. These testimonies encouraged me and helped me overcome any doubts I may have had about this being possible. By the time I was ready to start, I was excited to see what was going to happen. It felt like I was about to discover some new side of God.

At the time, I had started online classes at Dallas Theological Seminary, and I had nothing else to do but focus on school. It seemed like the perfect time, so I selected a day—May 25, 2020—and committed to it. I'd started a vegan diet on June 17, 2019, which I believe helped me go into the fast. And I didn't drink coffee at that time, so I didn't have to worry about caffeine headaches, which are a typical withdrawal symptom within the first two or three days of a fast (though they usually subside after that).

I had read stories of people encountering Jesus during fasts, and my heart was crying out, "God, I want to know more of you. I don't know what's going to happen to me in this fast, but even if I die, I know my heart is in the right place. I am seeking you, and I know where I'm going." In my faith, I had confidence that everything was going to be OK. That was my attitude as I began the fast, and it carried me through those difficult early days.

Now, I want to share with you what I personally experienced so you will have some idea of what to expect during your own fast. Later, we will break this down into more detail as I examine the different phases of fasting. In doing so, I want to help you in the same way that my friend Colin helped me by giving you a road map of the fasting journey so you can prepare your heart and your mind for what is to come.

Enduring the Ebbs and Flows

During the first few days of my fast, I had very little energy. All I wanted to do was lie down. Schoolwork kept my mind occupied, which helped, but other than a lack of energy, physically, I felt fine. I took up running as my exercise routine to stay physically fit. Within the first two weeks of the fast, I would feel great some days and jog an average of two miles.

There were some strange food withdrawal symptoms, but not in the way that I expected. I remember having a vivid dream about eating Oreos, but it felt like a nightmare. I woke up in a cold sweat, terrified that I had somehow broken my fast in the night. Since then, through many more fasts, I have learned that these kinds of food-related dreams are common about four or five days into a fast. It's just the body's natural mechanism for reminding us to eat.

When I woke up and realized that I hadn't actually broken my fast, it encouraged me and gave me a boost. My mouth was really dry, so I had a nice glass of water, which was refreshing, and I was strengthened to continue past day five.

There are ebbs and flows to fasting, and you have to be prepared for that. Some days, I felt like absolute garbage. My mind was cloudy, I couldn't focus, and I didn't want to get out of bed. But other days, I felt great—energized and peaceful. You have to be ready for the occasional battle, trusting that they don't last forever.

One struggle I didn't anticipate was boredom. So much of our time is consumed with food—thinking about food, planning meals, buying food, consuming it, cleaning dishes afterward—that during a fast, you find you have a lot of extra free time. At first, I didn't know what to do with this additional time. I'd already made the decision to cut out television and video games. I had schoolwork, but it didn't take up more than a few hours a week. I tried to fill the extra time with Bible reading and prayer, but my old prayer routine became a struggle as I found it harder to focus.

I had a desire to spend time with Jesus in prayer, and it was part of my daily routine. I would get out of bed, kneel in my bedroom, read my Bible, and pray. However, this routine became increasingly difficult during the fast. Initially, I forced myself to do it anyway, but it just didn't feel right. Eventually, I realized that maybe God was trying to show me something.

Maybe He wanted me to learn that there are different ways to spend time with Him. Maybe I needed to break my routine. I didn't have to be on my knees in my bedroom. I could go outside onto the side porch at my parent's house, watch the sun rise, listen to the birds, and talk to Jesus as if He were sitting right beside me. I could read one Bible verse and meditate on it for days. It may seem like a small thing, but this realization had a profound effect on my spiritual life. Jesus just wanted to spend time with me. He didn't need me to approach Him in some specific way, in some specific posture, with some rigid routine.

He used this first fast to show me the freedom we have in approaching Him, as 2 Corinthians 3:17 says, "Now the Lord is the Spirit, and where the Spirit of the Lord is, there is freedom." Jesus was freeing me from the spirit of religion.

For most of my life, when I approached Jesus, it was to request something. Through the fasting process, Jesus showed me that I could just sit with Him. He enjoys my company. I don't need to do anything. I don't need to perform, say eloquent prayers, or earn my way into his presence. All I have to do is posture my heart and mind toward Him and intentionally meet with Him. The more I did this, the more He filled me with His love. I began to understand His heart, and I started caring less about myself and wanting more of what He wanted.

As I went deeper into the fast, I began to experience bursts of energy at night. I would spend that time doing pushups, sit-ups, and light dumbbell exercises—just enough to get my body moving. I felt good. My blood was flowing, and the lethargy was gone. I actually felt worse when I was lying in bed.

I also began to experience a remarkable mental clarity. I could focus better in class, and writing papers became easier as my thoughts flowed more naturally. My communication sharpened, and all my senses seemed heightened. My eyesight and hearing improved, and I could even taste water more vividly. My sense of smell became so acute that I could detect the body odor of people around me, whether they had showered or not, which sometimes made being in close quarters quite challenging. In a nonfasted state, our natural senses are not as sharp, and we likely don't notice the odors of others unless they are wearing strong perfume, but I could now smell even a light perfume from several rows away.

I reached a point during the fast where the presence of food didn't affect me. The smell of food, even cooking it, becomes almost pleasurable. It's as if I was experiencing the food in a different way without feeling the temptation to eat it. I thought, *This smells good*, but I didn't feel hungry. The hunger ceased, allowing me to push through the temptations of food more easily.

I required less sleep, as my body wasn't burdened with digesting food. During the days when I felt terrible, I now understand that my body was using stored fat and other impurities as fuel. These down days were a sign that my body was detoxifying. Once the toxins were processed, I would feel a surge of energy and overall improvement over the next one to three days. This cycle tends to repeat itself throughout fasts I've completed that were fourteen to forty days.

This process is not just physical but also spiritual. The spiritual side has to do with the thoughts and emotions that come up during the fast. It requires a constant dying to self (getting frustrated because you can't eat), your wants (to eat), and your desires (not wanting to confront hard thoughts and emotions).

I share this to encourage you not to quit when you feel awful, especially during the first few days of fasting. If you've never fasted for more than a day or two, it can be a challenging new experience that requires discipline and effort. It's important to settle your heart and let the Holy Spirit guide you through it. God will provide the grace you need to persevere.

When I felt like quitting, particularly after day five when I had that vivid dream about eating, I would call my friend Colin for support. He advised me to break the fast into manageable time frames. My initial goal was to reach five days, which was the longest I had ever fasted. After achieving that, I aimed for ten to twelve days, based on

Colin's encouragement that I would start to feel better around that time. This approach helped me stay focused and committed to the fast.

There were numerous moments when I doubted my ability to continue. I often thought, *I'll just make it to day ten and then call it quits.* I was ready to be satisfied with that and attempt a longer fast some other time. Thankfully, Colin kept encouraging me, saying, "It's going to be worth it, man. Just keep going. Try to go another day." This advice helped me persevere. I started taking it one day at a time.

One of the more challenging aspects of that first fast was the difficulty sleeping. My body simply didn't need as much rest, so I averaged around four hours of sleep a night, especially from days ten to twenty-one. And sleep wasn't continuous; I frequently woke up to use the restroom because I was staying well-hydrated, drinking lots of water. At that time, I was drinking spring water, specifically Ice Mountain, a brand that is widely available in the Chicago area. However, after day eighteen, drinking this water became uncomfortable. It began to taste bitter and felt scratchy in my throat.

Later, I learned that the minerals in spring water can affect its flavor and make it rougher to drink during a long fast. Distilled water, which is pure H_2O with all minerals removed, was much smoother and easier to drink as the fast progressed. Therefore, I recommend starting with distilled water and sticking with it throughout the fast to avoid any discomfort or issues.

Switching to distilled water, however, caused an unexpected reaction in my body. I started having loose bowel movements after being constipated up to that point. This worried me, making me think something was wrong. I've learned it helps to stay consistent with the same type (distilled, spring, alkaline) and brand of water during the fast.

This experience taught me that, during a first fast, it's common to become overly focused on physical symptoms. It's important to wage a mental and spiritual battle, focusing on Jesus and not on physical conditions. Don't worry about your weight, blood pressure, or bowel movements. Avoid weighing yourself or getting caught up in the physical changes, challenges, and discomforts that will inevitably come up. The enemy will try to use these things to cause fear and tempt you to quit.

The purpose of fasting is not physical but spiritual growth. It's an opportunity to deepen your hunger for Jesus, enhance your spiritual hearing, and spend more time in prayer and reading the Bible. Use the time you would normally spend preparing and eating food to engage in activities that draw you closer to God: read edifying books, listen to podcasts, go on a prayer walk, pray for someone, play worship music, take a nap, watch a sermon, attend small groups and prayer nights at church, participate in family activities.

Or use the money you would normally spend on food for yourself and help out a family in need. Bring food to a homeless person and share the gospel. Your senses and mind will become incredibly sharp, almost like a supercomputer, allowing you to absorb vast amounts of information. Use this heightened focus to seek the Lord, study the Bible, journal, and do things that build you up spiritually.

If you experience ailments or side effects, or if you find yourself unsure about what's happening to your body, know that you're going to be OK. I'm not a doctor, but I can tell you that having someone who has gone through fasting or consulting a doctor who understands fasting can be very helpful. However, be aware that many doctors may not have experience with fasting.

Preparation and Timing Are Key

Preparation and timing are key to a successful fast. During my journey, I was fortunate to have a block of time where I only needed to focus on school and the fast. I didn't have the responsibilities of a family, which can create challenges and significantly impact the fasting experience.

If you have a spouse or children, they will inevitably feel the effects of your fast. Your partner doesn't have to fast with you, but their understanding and support are important. It can be challenging if your spouse has never fasted and doesn't understand what you're going through, and this can sometimes lead to discouragement. For example, I know some people who stopped their fast because their spouse was too stressed or uncomfortable with the situation.

Fasting can create a sense of isolation, especially socially, because being around people who are eating can be difficult. You might face questions like, "Why aren't you eating?" These moments can be challenging, especially during your first fast. It's important to be sensitive to the posture of your heart and avoid prideful sharing. The Bible advises against fasting publicly to show off, as the Pharisees did. Their intention was to appear holy. As long as your intention is not to show off but to stay humble, you can navigate these social situations appropriately. If you feel even a hint of pride, it's better to keep your fast private, saying something like, "I'm just not eating at the moment," or "It's something personal between me and the Lord."

Eventually, you might become comfortable enough to talk about your fast without pride, which can become a way to witness and help others grow closer to Jesus. That's where my heart is now, and it's why I'm writing this book. It's not about drawing attention to myself or showing off my fasting achievements. It's about sharing what the Lord has done in me through fasting, what I've learned, and how He can work in your life through the power of fasting. I hope to prepare you for the various challenges you might face and help you grow closer to Jesus through your own fasting journey.

However, after twenty-one days, the fast can become more challenging, primarily from a mental and spiritual warfare perspective. Physically, there will be days when you will not have energy other than to lie down. Emotionally, there will be times of feeling lonely and depressed. It's important to plan ahead of time and make sure you keep an open schedule. I highly recommend taking a break from work if possible. One of the most powerful things you can do is take time off specifically for fasting. When was the last time you heard someone say, "I'm going to take off work so I can fast to get closer to Jesus"?

If you can take a month off for a thirty-day fast, or even two months for a forty-day fast followed by forty days of breaking the fast, do it. Rent an Airbnb or find a friend with a cabin to retreat to. Jesus will honor the fact you are sacrificing food, time, finances, family, friendships, and your desires to spend time with Him. It will be life-changing.

In order to avoid temptation, it can be helpful to clear your cabinets of food before starting the fast. I've found that having no food at home reduces the temptation to break the fast. Whatever the case, be prepared to push through the challenges with the mentality of seeking more of the Lord. Don't let "breaking the fast early" be an option, except in the most dire of circumstances.

Having a supportive community also helps. Attending prayer nights, church services, or worship gatherings where food isn't present can be beneficial. Engaging in or leading Bible studies can provide support and focus.

An Obstacle I Couldn't Overcome

Around day twenty-one or twenty-two of my first fast, I experienced a breakout on my skin. Small red dots appeared on my left side, around my ribs, and they were itchy. My friend Colin had never experienced this, so I began to feel concerned. I wondered if it was serious, if it was permanent, and if it was a sign to stop. These concerns consumed my thoughts and prayers.

Physical ailments can manifest in various ways during a fast, such as acid reflux, headaches, nausea, dizziness, fainting, vomiting, body aches, muscle twitching, fatigue, a fluctuating heart rate, diarrhea, constipation, skin rashes, feeling cold, dry mouth, white coating on the tongue, various side effects from getting off medication, or weakness. I've experienced lightheadedness and weakness myself. Mild physical ailments should never be a reason to break a fast. However, my rash worsened, spreading to my right side and then to the middle of my stomach. By day twenty-three, it became severe.

I considered using external treatments like oil or cream and even researched remedies. Some people suggested coconut oil. I applied coconut oil and tried to get some sun for vitamin D, but these actions only worsened the condition. The itching became unbearable. This skin issue ultimately led me to break the fast. Despite feeling mentally and physically fine otherwise, the rash was an obstacle I couldn't overcome. I remember rollerblading outside around day twenty-two, which likely added stress to my body and accelerated the breakout. In hindsight, I wouldn't recommend such intense physical activities during a fast.

Eventually, I shared my condition with my parents, and they advised me to break the fast. This experience taught me valuable lessons, which I share to help others avoid similar mistakes. If you encounter physical issues during your fast, consider seeking medical advice and avoid self-treating in ways that might exacerbate the problem.

Since then, I have discovered that skin breakouts are a normal part of the process for some people. These breakouts, which can appear as tiny red dots or eczema-like patches, are a byproduct of the increase of ketones in the body and the body expelling toxins. I panicked when I experienced this during my first fast, but I know now that these symptoms are temporary. After eventually completing several other fasts over thirty days, I noticed these skin breakouts began to subside. I also learned in this journey of fasting that it may take several long fasts for the body to heal and detox all the junk inside.

A friend of mine who completed a forty-day fast experienced similar breakouts and was informed by her doctor that it was related to ketosis. Ketosis, a state where the body uses fat as fuel, often causes skin issues because of the excess ketones and increased acidity in the blood. This revelation helped me understand my own experience. Instead of using anti-itch creams, I recommend enduring the discomfort naturally. Wear a T-shirt and gently rub the affected areas to alleviate itchiness.

Lightheadedness is another common issue during extended fasts. It's important to take your time when getting up from a lying or sitting position. Sit up slowly, count to ten, and let the blood flow to your brain before standing. If you feel lightheaded, lean on something or sit down immediately to avoid fainting. This adjustment period is important to prevent accidents.

These physical symptoms, while challenging, are part of the fasting journey. They should not cause panic or fear but should be anticipated and managed calmly. Focusing on Jesus and maintaining a spiritual mindset can help you navigate these challenges. That can be as simple as lying down for a few minutes and praying, "Jesus, I can't do this on my own. Give me strength and grace." Take a few deep breaths. You will feel a supernatural strength and peace overcome you.

Exercise during fasting should be gentle and manageable. While vigorous activities like running are not recommended, walking can be beneficial. Walking for an hour or two daily, even at a slow pace, can improve your mood and energy levels. It provides fresh air and movement, and it helps you feel less lethargic.

Fasting with Confidence and Peace

Ultimately, these insights are meant to prepare you for the physical aspects of fasting so you can remain focused on the spiritual journey. By understanding and managing these symptoms, you can continue to fast with confidence and peace, knowing that they are normal parts of the process.

Emotionally, after about ten days of fasting, you'll start feeling more levelheaded and calmer. Anxiety diminishes, and you may experience a serene sense of closeness to Jesus. This is because fasting cleanses the body, the temple of God (1 Corinthians 6:19–20), allowing the Holy Spirit to dwell within you more prominently (1 Corinthians 3:16). You become more attuned to the Holy Spirit's guidance, exhibiting the fruits that are love, peace, patience, kindness, goodness, gentleness, faithfulness, and self-control (Galatians 5:22). Earthly concerns lose their grip; your focus shifts solely to spending time with Jesus (Colossians 3:1–2). Achievements and material pursuits seem less significant compared to the sweet, intimate relationship with the Holy Spirit.

However, spiritual warfare can make you feel edgy. The enemy often attempts to disrupt your fast. For example, you might encounter unexpected temptations like free pizza at work on the second day of your fast or a bowl of your favorite chocolates appearing in your apartment lobby. These occurrences are surprisingly common and serve as distractions aimed at breaking your fast.

In my own experience, on the first day of a long fast, someone put a bowl of my favorite chocolate, Reese's, in the elevator lobby, so every time I left or returned to my apartment, I would pass by the bowl. Another time, on the third or fourth day of a different fast, I encountered free donuts being handed out at a mail center, a highly unusual event. Such temptations are not coincidences; they are deliberate attempts to deter you from fasting.

Understanding these challenges is vital to your success. Recognizing them as spiritual warfare equips you with the wisdom to resist. You may feel more irritable, quick to anger, or emotionally sensitive during a fast. These reactions could be your flesh; outside attacks of the enemy; manifestations of demonic oppression; underlying issues like pride, depression, anxiety, selfishness, fear, insecurity, lust, control, hatred, or unforgiveness; emotional or mental trauma; addictions; or other strongholds that fasting brings to the surface for purification.

When you feel irritable during a fast, take a moment and pray, "Jesus, why do I feel this way? Where is this coming from?" Then listen. Some of the most powerful moments in the fast happen when you take time to self-reflect with Jesus, talk to Him, and journal what's going on. Once He reveals the root cause, ask Jesus what He wants to do with it. Give it to Him and ask Him what He is giving you in return. This simple process allows for inner healing.

Fasting acts as a mirror, prompting deep self-reflection. I remember during my first fast, I realized how much anger and pride I harbored. I didn't like talking to people, I was selfish, and I often spoke harshly to my parents, even when they were just checking in on me. This made me question my reactions and led to a revelation: many of my emotional responses stemmed from childhood wounds.

As a child, I didn't know how to process my parents' approach to parenting, and I internalized these feelings. During the fast, these suppressed emotions resurfaced. So when my parents innocently asked how I was doing, my irritated response came from a place of unresolved childhood hurt. Fasting highlighted these wounds and allowed me to reflect and understand their origins. This led to moments of vulnerability with my parents, where I apologized and explained my reactions, which brought about inner healing and deliverance.

Throughout the fast, similar challenges emerged. The enemy often uses close loved ones to cause division or discourage you. For example, someone you admire, like a mentor or pastor, might criticize your fasting, calling you foolish. Such moments are tactics to distract you from focusing on Jesus. People may genuinely care for you and have good intentions, but the enemy could use that as a weapon.

I experienced the enemy's attempts to use my family to derail my fast, which made me feel disconnected from the Lord. However, by bringing these struggles to the Lord, I allowed Him to purify my heart and change me. If you don't address these issues with the Lord's help, the enemy can cause significant damage. I share this not to instill fear but to increase awareness. The enemy will try everything to prevent you from getting closer to the Lord, receiving revelations, and experiencing life-changing transformations through fasting.

Despite these challenges, there is supernatural protection and strength from the Lord. Jesus was also tempted (Matthew 4:1; Hebrews 4:15), but He refused to sin, and so can you. Praying, quoting Scriptures, and spending time with Jesus will strengthen you for these battles.

What I Learned from My First Fast

In my first journey, I initially focused on the physical aspects rather than the spiritual. Although I managed to complete my schoolwork with sharp focus, my answered prayers and spiritual growth became clearer as I continued.

I was initially quite irritable, but the Lord challenged me to change my heart and transform my anger and hatred into love. For example, when I ran, He urged me to pray for every person I passed. This practice helped me develop a heart of love. Through fasting, I learned to let go of pride and selfishness and embrace a more compassionate attitude toward others.

Over time, the Lord began to give me *His* heart for people, instilling in me a deep desire to share the gospel, His love, and His truth with others. This awakening ignited a fire within me because I realized the eternal significance of people's souls. Understanding that every person is destined for either heaven or hell, I felt compelled to share the message of Jesus Christ, who offers salvation through faith because of His sacrifice on the cross.

I used to lack the boldness to share openly. However, the fast revealed aspects of myself I hadn't seen before—the ugliness, the anger, fear of man, fear of rejection, and selfishness. This introspection led to significant inner healing and deliverance. When my heart changed, I learned to die to self, to help others, and to not live a self-centered life. These were the fruits of the fast, answers to prayer, and the Lord's voice guiding me.

Interestingly, I didn't hear or see much during the fast itself because of the burden and weight of the journey. It felt like going through a refining fire. The real fruits and answers appeared after the fast. There was no specific time frame for these answers; they came when the Lord willed it.

About a month after that first fast, God confirmed His call on my life. I met a friend who introduced me to his uncle, a man known for his prophetic prayers. Although I was cautious and wanted to test this experience as the Bible advises, I felt it was an open door from the Lord. The uncle, who knew nothing about me, prayed for me and prophesied that God would use me to share the gospel in other countries. This prophecy confirmed what I had heard before from a pastor's wife in the Philippines who had prophesied similarly over me.

I believe this confirmation was a fruit of the fast, reassuring me of God's plans for my life. My steps were being directed clearly, a testament to the power of fasting and seeking the Lord earnestly.

Since then, almost every time I've undertaken a long consecrated fast, I've experienced moments where the Lord speaks to me through people who know nothing about my situation. These individuals become His mouthpieces, conveying messages that align perfectly with what I'm going through and what I'm seeking. The messages always conform to biblical teachings, and they often confirm something the Lord has already placed in my heart or revealed to me through a Bible verse. This confirmation is incredibly encouraging.

I believe everyone has access to this divine guidance. The Bible promises that the Lord is close to the brokenhearted and those who seek Him earnestly. Jeremiah 29:13 says, "You will seek me and find me when you seek me with all your heart." And Joel 2:12 says, "'Yet even now,' declares the Lord, 'return to me with all your heart, with fasting, with weeping, and with mourning.'"

Fasting, denying yourself the comfort of food—one of the greatest bodily needs—to put Jesus first is a powerful way to seek God with all your heart. By giving up food, you demonstrate your total commitment to seeking Him. In this posture of surrender, you will encounter the Lord. He will speak to you, give you visions, dreams, and direction, bring healing, clarify your calling, and bring revival to your life.

Each fasting journey is unique and dynamic, revealing new areas of freedom, highlighting new areas of bondage that need breaking, and uncovering generational iniquities that need to be addressed. There are certain issues in our lives that can only be resolved through this powerful spiritual discipline.

We're going to look more deeply at the phases of fasting soon, but before you begin your first fast, there are some things you can do to prepare for it. If you start your fast with the right planning, it will be easier to focus on the spiritual, overcome the inevitable ebbs and flows, avoid any discouragement from fasting, and get the most out of the experience to where you'll be able to walk through many life-changing, prolonged consecrated fasts of twenty-one- to forty days.

CHAPTER 5: TRAINING FOR A FAST

What's important to remember from my own experience with fasting is that everyone is different. Some people can dive right into a prolonged fast, but not everyone is built that way. For instance, my dad jumped straight into a forty-two-day fast after hearing about my experience. He didn't even tell me he was doing it until day thirty-eight.

While I believe anyone can potentially undertake a similar journey, I also understand that not everyone has the same opportunity, attitude, or drive. For many people, a training period may be necessary before beginning a prolonged fast. In fact, this training period can deepen your spiritual journey and strengthen you almost as much as the fast itself.

First of all, I encourage you to start training by changing your diet. This will help prepare your physical body, but more importantly, you need to prepare yourself spiritually. Spend time before your fast seeking the Lord with a genuine hunger to know Him more deeply, to grow, and allow Him to work in your life in ways you haven't experienced before.

Ask Jesus what He is putting on your heart. Is He leading you to a forty-day fast, a one-day fast each week, or just skipping one meal a day? While Jesus expects us to fast, the specifics can vary for each person. You may be unfamiliar with fasting, or you might find the idea of a forty-day fast overwhelming. That's OK. Take baby steps if you need to and don't feel bad about it. There is power in simply starting.

Baby Steps to a Full Fast

Changing your diet is an important first step to preparing for a long fast. Transitioning to a healthier diet will ease the fasting process. For example, as I explained in the introduction, I switched from a regular diet to vegetarian and then to a vegan diet, eating mostly fruits and vegetables. Preparing your body in this way makes the initial days of fasting easier. If you're a coffee drinker, wean yourself off coffee gradually, starting at least seven days before the fast, no longer drinking coffee three days before the fast, to prevent caffeine withdrawal headaches.

"Almost all fasting attempts fail through ignorance of the fact that with the beginning of the mucusless diet the old mucus is being excreted so much more forcibly until that person is absolutely clean and healthy."[34]

In other words, your body purges itself of years of poor eating, medication, diseases, and excess garbage within the body. The cleansing can become so intense it may feel as if you are dying. This causes many people to quit within the first few days of fasting and avoid it completely without ever experiencing the life-changing transformation spiritually, physically, mentally, and emotionally.

Therefore, if you have never been on a diet, stopped eating meat, stopped drinking coffee, skipped a meal, or stopped taking medication, it may be necessary to make small changes to your diet and lifestyle before embarking on a prolonged fast. This is where I recommend following Daniel's diet. Even in these small changes, while it isn't technically fasting, God sees the posture of your heart and will reward these changes in your life. There's still wisdom, knowledge, and revelation to be gained in the preparation.

Next, incorporate some light exercise. If you're not used to running, start by walking two to three miles a day, then gradually begin jogging. Exercise helps your body get rid of junk, such as fat, and toxins, and improves your overall health. This physical activity helps prepare your body for fasting because, in a fast, there is an acceleration of your body removing garbage and purifying the blood. This process can make you feel sick for several days at the beginning of a fast. Physically preparing will help ease some of these symptoms during the fast.

Once your diet is stable (for example, I was on a vegan diet for over eleven months before any prolonged fast over twenty-one days), you can begin taking baby steps into fasting. For example, you might start by skipping your morning meal once a week for a month, then increase it to three times a week. Then start choosing to eat only one healthy meal a day for dinner. Do this once a week and build up to multiple times a week. Gradually, aim for a twenty-four-hour fast once or twice a week, and then build up to two consecutive days per week. Eventually, you can aim for three days per week, either consecutively or every other day.

By taking these steps, you will progressively build your capacity for longer fasts while also deepening your spiritual journey. After that, several months later or the following year, if you feel ready to attempt a longer fast, this gradual preparation will help you get started.

The point is to take baby steps to build up your endurance and strength. This method prepares you for a long fast, just as you would train for a marathon or study for a big exam. You dedicate time each day to prepare, and eventually, you're ready to apply what you've learned.

Your training period can last as long as you need it to. You might decide that after a year of preparation, you're ready to attempt your first long fast at the beginning of the following year. If you are healthy, exercise daily, and if you have fasted before, you may be able to progress faster into a long fast. You may even jump right into a prolonged fast without preparation. This is between you and the Lord.

Remember, multiple attempts might be necessary. Training for a fast often involves some trial and error, and that's OK. Don't beat yourself up over it. You might aim for a long fast but only manage four days before needing to stop. That's still a significant achievement. Each attempt is valuable, and God sees the intent of your heart. The enemy might try to discourage you by highlighting your perceived failures, but remind yourself that seeking the Lord and attempting to fast is already a victory.

For example, there were times when I felt led to do a long fast but struggled to get past day three because of cravings. Even though I gave in to the cravings and ate, I didn't beat myself up. I restarted and gradually managed to go longer. As I said, it's similar to training for a marathon. You might attempt to run the full distance but need to stop after a few miles. So you try again another day, and even if you walk part of the distance, you're still successfully working toward your goal.

Sometimes, even with perfect preparation, a fast still feels incredibly difficult. Other times, with God's grace, even a forty-day fast might feel surprisingly easy. It's difficult to set exact expectations or guarantee success. The steps I share are practical tips I've learned, which I wish I had known earlier. They provide a framework to help you on your journey.

The good news is there will always be a meaningful outcome to your fast, even if it's not immediately visible. Every fasting story in the Bible had an outcome. The spiritual journey of fasting has lasting effects, sometimes seen in your lifetime or perhaps in your children's lifetimes. Moses partook in two forty-day fasts, and God told Moses he would lead them to the Promised Land. Moses died before he could get a chance to enter the Promised Land, but the next generation of Israelites entered the Promised Land (Deuteronomy 34:4–5). The point being that each step away from food will bring you a step closer to Jesus.

Gathering Support

It's important to have someone who has gone through a long fast or has experience with fasting to support you, especially for your first time. You need both spiritual encouragement *and* practical advice.

From a physical standpoint, it's wise to inform your doctor about your plans, even though you might face pushback since many doctors and people in general find the idea of fasting extreme. Dr. Arnold Ehert warns of this as well: "Neither fasting nor the fruit diet have been accepted by the medical authorities nor have they been used by others in strict accordance with the condition of the patient; yet when properly combined as a 'systematic cleansing', the treatment has been remarkably successful and satisfactory."[35]

Their lack of understanding often focuses only on the physical aspects, not considering the spiritual journey you're undertaking. Even so, if it gives you peace of mind, then alerting your doctor is a good thing, especially if you have existing health conditions or are on medication. If you have never had health troubles, you may not need to tell a doctor but rather only someone who has done a prolonged fast.

The best way to mentally prepare for a fast is to gather resources on topics you want to explore or grow in during the fast. This may include books on fasting or other Bible topics. Prepare these materials in advance so you have them ready.

The fasting period involves a lot of spiritual warfare, so plan ahead with edifying resources. Podcasts, spiritually uplifting music, and faith-based movies and shows like *The Chosen* can support your spiritual growth during this time. Avoid any content that might negatively impact your spiritual journey, such as movies with sinful or demonic content or music with crude lyrics, as they can interfere with the fast. Cut out social media, news, and the internet, and even put a pause on relationships that are negatively impacting you. Don't seek out pleasure or anything stimulating during the fast.

It's a good idea to keep a journal during your fast, especially if you enjoy writing. It's also helpful to have someone to talk to during the fast. Although fasting should be done in a humble and private manner, sharing your journey with a trusted friend, mentor, or partner doesn't violate the principle of fasting in secret. The key is the posture of your heart. If you're sharing to seek attention or validation, you're missing the point. The Bible criticizes the religious hypocrites who fasted publicly for self-righteous reasons (Matthew 6:16). However, sharing with a supportive friend for mutual encouragement is different, and God sees the intent of your heart.

Finally, this book is designed to offer the guidance and support you might need during your fast, so feel free to return here as often as you want. Whatever you do, be aware of potential discouragement, pushback, and resistance during your fast, especially from people who don't understand the spiritual aspect of this journey. The enemy will try to discourage you in a lot of different ways, but the purpose of your fast is to grow closer to Jesus and strengthen your faith. No fasting attempt is ever a failure but only a stepping stone to growth. Jesus loves it, sees it, acknowledges all of it, and will be there with you every step of the way. That is guaranteed!

Here is an encouraging testimony from my mom's experience:

> Dear brothers and sisters in Christ,
>
> After I fasted for eighteen days, my unbelief was driven away. I am experiencing salvation for the body and the soul. The body is saved from sickness as the soul becomes saved from sin.
>
> For me, fasting is a spiritual discipline that helps me grow in faith. Fasting helped me to posture my heart in humility toward God. Jesus tells

us to pray and fast quietly, humbly, and without pride. While fasting, I spent more time in prayer and God's word. Fasting gave me freedom from weakness; it gave me strength, healed me from the inside out, and helped me to make the necessary changes, awakening fresh life in me.

I waited for God in the fast for a breakthrough to do the impossible in and through me. I'm choosing to believe that's true. He set me free from bondage. After fasting, I can say no to things that distract me mentally, physically, emotionally, and spiritually. I'm empowered with strength and peace.

I admit I need more fasting and prayer for miracles, but here I am again, delivered from my tendency toward anxiety and worry. God showed me that He fights for me. I have to press on toward the goal of winning the prize for which He called me and the ability to persevere. Fasting was hard, but the Holy Ghost gave me the strength and determination to keep moving forward. I learned the power of perseverance. I'm free from worrying and trying so hard to work everything out in my strength. It has helped me to trust more of the Scriptures. I am more thankful for the abundance of blessings and goodness already stored up, for wisdom and the perspective to see my sin as God sees it, and He gave me the strength to overcome sin by His grace.

—*Estera Trinca Sr.*

CHAPTER 6: BEGINNING A FAST

So *when* should you begin your fast, and how should you go about selecting a starting date? Sometimes, the beginning of a fast may coincide with things that are happening in your life.

In Acts 9:1–19, we read about the profound conversion experience of Saul (who, after his encounter with Jesus, became Paul). Notably, in verse 9, it says that Saul was without sight for three days and neither ate nor drank. This period of fasting wasn't a decision Saul made on his own. Rather, it was a product of his encounter with Jesus.

Numerous biblical stories highlight different reasons for fasting: Nehemiah fasted for the rebuilding of Jerusalem, Daniel fasted for wisdom and consecration, and Moses and Elijah fasted to draw near to God. In these instances, fasting was often a deliberate decision to seek something specific from God. However, it's important to remember that fasting is not a transactional act, as if we were saying, "God, I will fast, and in return, you will do something for me." Rather, fasting should always be chiefly a means to seek God's will and express a deep hunger for His presence.

Saul had extensive knowledge of Old Testament Scriptures as a result of his rigorous religious education, and he believed he was serving God by persecuting the followers of Jesus because, before his encounter with Jesus, he didn't believe Jesus was the Messiah.

He was a zealous, religious man who was convinced that his actions were righteous. Acts 9:1 depicts Saul's fervor, detailing his threats and acts of violence. He sought permission from the high priest to arrest anyone who followed Jesus, and in doing so, he believed he was stamping out heresy.

This should prompt us to reflect on how many of us, confident in our religious activities and understanding, might be blind to our own misguided efforts. Saul's dramatic encounter with Jesus on the road to Damascus led to a revelation of his spiritual blindness. Jesus's question, "Why are you persecuting me?" and the subsequent blinding light brought Saul to his knees, both literally and metaphorically.

For three days, Saul experienced a forced fast, unable to see, eat, or drink. This period symbolizes a divine intervention where God brings a person to a point of complete surrender, stripping away self-reliance and leading them to seek Him wholeheartedly. Saul's fasting was not a planned spiritual discipline but a natural outcome of his life-altering experience.

During this time, God spoke to a believer named Ananias and instructed him to go to Saul and deliver a message. When Ananias laid hands on Saul, something like scales fell from Saul's eyes, and he regained his sight. He then rose, was baptized, and was filled with the Holy Spirit. This sequence of events demonstrates that Saul's conversion and subsequent fast were integral to his spiritual awakening and salvation.

Saul's story teaches us that fasting can be a profound *response* to an encounter with God, one that signifies total surrender and a deep desire to align with His will. Rather than being a means to an end, it becomes a powerful act of worship and submission to God's sovereignty.

Indeed, when you encounter the Lord, it often requires time to process what has happened. One effective way to do this is through fasting. Saul fasted because he was likely still processing the profound experience he had just had on the road to Damascus. The

Scripture notes that, after this period, when he finally took food, he was strengthened.

On the flip side, it's important to remember that the flesh will never want to fast. Food is the greatest stronghold, especially in America, a land of abundance. Have you noticed that, even at the mere thought of fasting, even now while you're reading this, you can come up with all types of excuses for not fasting: "My spouse wouldn't want me to! I have to work! I'm afraid of dying! I'm sick! I need my cup of coffee! I'm too skinny! I love eating! I can't miss a meal! God will have grace if I don't! My pastor or church doesn't fast! It's too hard! I need more information! I'll wait until next year! God needs to give me a sign!"

If you are waiting for a perfect time to start, you may never end up fasting. You may never encounter biblical or personal circumstances that require or force you to fast. There will rarely ever be a convenient time to fast. In life, food and distractions will always surround you. You simply have to decide to start and press through. The flesh is weak, but the spirit is willing (Matthew 26:41). Here's your confirmation: You need to fast. Begin this walk today by turning away from food and taking steps to get closer to Jesus through fasting.

Deciding the Duration of Your Fast

The duration of your fast may be uncertain, and it may require a daily pursuit of God. In Saul's case, his fast ended when God sent Ananias to deliver a message, heal him, and open his eyes. The moment of healing marked the end of his fast, showing that it was actually God who had ordained the length and purpose of his fast.

The Holy Spirit might prompt you to fast for a specific period, such as fourteen days, or to start a fast without a specific number of days and then provide further clarity or answers during the journey. Other times, the Holy Spirit will lead you to fast until you experience a breakthrough. However, as I said before, fasting should be approached with a heart seeking God, not as a means to gain something. Don't stop a fast early just because you got what you wanted out of it. For example, you might commit to a twenty-one-day fast seeking direction from God, and even if you receive clarity on day two, you should continue fasting out of gratitude and a desire to honor your commitment. This demonstrates a posture of thankfulness and a continuous hunger for more of God.

Remember, the primary reason for fasting should always be a deep love for Jesus and a desire to grow closer to Him. Under the new covenant in Jesus, all acts of devotion are done in faith and meant to be rooted in love for Him (James 2:18). Fasting, therefore, should be a response to His sacrifice and love, driven by a desire to know Him more intimately and to seek His will. It should not be about adhering to strict religious rules or asceticism, but about deepening your relationship with God.

As I mentioned earlier, sharing your fast with other people can be a delicate matter. Early in your spiritual journey, it might be wise to keep your fasting private to avoid pride or seeking validation from others. Fasting is, after all, a personal act between you and God when done with the right heart posture. Over time, as your relationship with Jesus matures and your humility grows, you may be able to talk about your fasting with the right attitude.

You may never feel the need to tell anyone about completing a forty-day fast, and that's perfectly fine. The point, if you do share, is to glorify Jesus and what He has done in your life through the fasting journey, inspiring others to grow in their hunger for Him. If this book has impacted you and you want others to experience the same, consider giving it to them as a gift.

Personally, it took me four years to begin writing about my fasting journey because I knew my intent had to be pure, not seeking attention for myself but aiming to share the knowledge and revelations

God has shown me. God started confirming it through other people telling me to write about fasting. Eventually, He gave me peace to begin. My goal now is to help others like you on your journey to encounter Him. Examine the intent of your heart when sharing about your fast. Are you looking for guidance, to share the impact it's had in your life, to point people to Jesus? Or are you trying to boast and bring glory to yourself?

Get Ready for a Challenge

Reflecting on my own experience in my first fast, I aimed for a forty-day fast but was humbled by God to complete only twenty-five days. Another attempt resulted in a fourteen-day fast. It took me over a period of four years to finally complete a forty-day fast. Through these experiences, I learned that fasting is about dying to self, purifying the heart, and seeking more of God. Sometimes, pride sets unrealistic goals, but Jesus will guide you to a length that truly benefits your spiritual growth.

Ultimately, the intent and posture of your heart should determine when you start the fast, as well as the length of your fast. It's a personal decision between you and Jesus, rooted in a sincere desire to grow closer to Him. If you're unsure about the duration, start with a hunger to grow and seek God, and He will make the path clear. You might find peace at a certain point, or you might continue to the full length you initially felt led to. However, the duration can vary based on what God places on your heart.

I've learned that having a burden for something can be powerful. Whether it's a desire for change in your marriage, healing in your body, a new hunger for Jesus, freedom from addictions, reformation in the American church, or revival in the nation, the deeper the burden, the stronger your resolve. This desire will help you overcome the temptations to give up and push through the challenges of fasting. The key is the intent of your heart and your desire to grow closer to Jesus. Whether you're seeking to know if God is real, need healing—physical or spiritual—or are facing deeply rooted struggles, each fast will draw you closer to God and transform you to become more like Him.

Nick Thummel, a friend of mine, explains his experience:

> This was my first prolonged fast (twenty-eight days). I had some fear of failure, not wanting to fall short of forty days. God gave me peace to start and not worry about the end destination. The first few days were the hardest. Massive headaches, nausea, and low energy. By day three or four, it got better. Day six to seven was new territory, and I hit a new wall of going further than my body had ever gone.
>
> During these days, it was like a roller coaster. There were times of clarity and intimacy with Jesus and times of feeling low, hurting, and distant from Him. It helped me to take it one day at a time and not think about the future. I struggled to stay focused in prayer, and there were spiritual battles that tried to intrude into my intimacy with the Lord.
>
> Remembering that the fast was a prayer in itself was helpful. By weeks three to four of the fast, I had gotten into a routine. Having a mindset of doing the fast, walking the steps, and reminding myself of Jesus and His focus on the mission kept me pushing through. I wanted to finish the fast when I was in a strong place, so even though I hadn't reached forty days, I prayed and had peace. I didn't want it to be about days or time. I didn't battle any guilt or shame for not completing forty days.

CHAPTER 7: THE FOUR PHASES OF FASTING

In his books on fasting, Franklin Hall breaks down fasting into a number of phases. While I agree with some of his ideas, my own experiences and research differ somewhat. However, it's important to remember that fasting phases are flexible and not set in stone. What I describe in this chapter is intended to serve as a guide to help you understand what you *might* experience physically, mentally, emotionally, and spiritually over the course of a prolonged fast. Everyone's experience can vary, but I want to provide awareness and support throughout your journey.

Phase One: Days One to Five

I define phase one as the first five days of fasting. Most people start and quit within the first five days. This period of time requires your full commitment and effort to avoid quitting the fast early. The difficulty level depends in large part on your diet prior to the fast, if you've been preparing through shorter fasts, and your physical health before the fast. If you abruptly switch from a poor diet of junk food or a diet rich in meats and seasonings to fasting, these first five days can be extremely tough. It could also be potentially harmful if you've been on medication for the majority of your life and stop taking it completely.

During this time, your body goes through intense detoxification, especially if you were consuming junk food, meat, alcohol, caffeine, medicine, and drugs regularly. You might experience severe headaches, nausea, vomiting, and general discomfort. As your body transitions from using glucose to entering ketosis, where it starts using stored fat for energy, you'll likely face intense cravings and may even dream about eating (like my Oreo nightmare).

During phase one, your thoughts will probably be consumed by food, which can lead to frustration. You're going to discover the hard way how much our lives revolve around eating—how it affects our time, money, thoughts, and even feelings. This increased awareness of the physical and spiritual aspects will deepen into other areas in later phases, but for now, you'll have to confront your dependence on food and see how powerfully it influences your daily life.

However, if you understand this and expect it, you can prepare yourself mentally and spiritually and stay committed despite these early challenges. To get through this phase, keep your mind busy in prayer, reading the Bible, and try to be active. That doesn't mean you have to be constantly in motion. Rest when you need to, and don't hesitate to sleep more if you feel unwell.

You will make this phase a lot easier on yourself if you prepare properly by gradually reducing your junk food, meat, alcohol, caffeine, medicine, and drug intake and adopting a clean diet *before* the fast. This will make the detox process quicker and less severe, which will make these first five days easier to handle.

Remember, feeling weak, sick, and tired is all part of the process. I'm focusing a lot on the physical because a person doing a prolonged fast for the first time has always been led by their carnal nature and may not have an understanding of the spiritual aspect. However, the most powerful thing you can do is pray anytime a challenge arises. Pray when you are tempted to eat. Pray when you want to quit. Pray when you feel all kinds of internal battles and physical weaknesses.

Bear in mind that many people quit during phase one, but if that happens to you, it's important to realize that no fast is a failure. Each attempt, regardless of its length, is a step toward spiritual growth. The intent behind your fast matters most, and even short fasts are an achievement. If you are reading this right now during your fast and have thoughts of quitting, my encouragement is to push through another day. It will get easier, and you will start to feel stronger. Take it one day at a time, pray, and watch your faith grow!

Powerful Prayer: "Holy Spirit, I yield to You. I can't do this on my own. Help me. Give me the strength to push through. Take my thoughts captive. Amen."

Phase Two: Days Six to Twelve

Phase two of fasting generally covers days six through twelve. During this phase, you'll notice that your hunger pangs start to decrease. This is because your body is adjusting to not eating at its usual times. If you're used to having three meals a day and have always done so your whole life, your body will initially protest when those meal times come around. This was particularly intense in phase one, where missing a meal felt very difficult.

In phase two, this becomes less intense, though your stomach might still growl at those regular meal times. When this happens, drinking water will help, and you can use these moments as reminders to pray and focus on your thoughts on Jesus. This is a good time to strengthen your connection with Jesus, replacing physical feeding with spiritual nourishment. Notice the wrestling of the physical body with the mind and heart. Your flesh wants to eat, but you want to hunger more for Jesus. I share this to bring awareness of what spiritual warfare looks like. Each time you subdue the fleshly desire to eat, you learn to yield to the Holy Spirit, which brings spiritual growth and sensitivity.

Dreams about food might occur as your body continues to adjust to the new routine. These dreams can seem like nightmares, but they are a normal part of the process. You may also experience some physical ailments, especially if you weren't in the best health to begin with. For those on medication, as we mentioned earlier, it's important to consult a doctor before starting a fast. Some people who abruptly stop taking their medication can experience withdrawal symptoms. It's better to gradually wean off medication before starting a fast to avoid intense side effects.

The detox process from phase one continues into phase two, but it might not be as intense. New symptoms could appear, or you might start feeling better as your body heals. A general symptom is a whitening of the tongue. You can lightly brush your tongue daily, but this whitening of the tongue is a sign your body is detoxing. This phase can have ups and downs, so it's important to listen to your body and adjust as needed. Generally, this phase is where the weakness of the body starts to leave.

Physical discomfort shouldn't be a reason to quit. In those tough moments, seek Jesus and pray for strength, and you may find that prayer gives you a burst of energy. It's important to keep your focus on the spiritual benefits of fasting, even when your faith feels weak and you are filled with doubt and frustration.

During this phase, you might feel tempted to give up, especially as the enemy tries to discourage you. Thoughts like *I've done enough* or *I can always restart* may surface. Do what you can to stay committed and continue seeking spiritual growth.

Around day ten, you'll notice improvements in your mental clarity and senses. Your mind will become sharper, and you'll begin to experience the benefits of fasting more clearly. This increased mental sharpness is a sign that your body and spirit are adapting well to the fast.

Powerful Prayer: "Jesus, You must increase, and I must decrease. Holy Spirit, purify my heart."

Phase Three: Days Thirteen to Twenty

Phase three of a prolonged fast usually lasts from day thirteen through day twenty. As I said, these phases aren't set in stone, and the length may vary by a day or two for different individuals. However, generally, at this point in the fast, cravings and hunger will largely (or entirely) subside, making this the "cruise control" phase.

By now, your body has adjusted to the fasting routine. If this is your first time reaching this phase, it's all going to feel quite new, so your focus will tend to be on the physical sensations you are experiencing because that's what is most apparent. Over time, through more fasting journeys, you'll gain deeper spiritual insights. At this phase, physically, your body is resting, healing, and cleansing. Detoxification continues, but it's typically less intense than in earlier phases.

However, minor physical challenges can still occur. You might feel unusually cold, have a fluctuating heart rate, or experience low energy levels. These are normal and should not cause panic or lead to quitting. The enemy may use these physical symptoms to instill fear and doubt.

Sleep requirements decrease during this phase because your body is using less energy. Your focus will sharpen, and your mental state will improve. You may notice enhanced senses—better eyesight, hearing, and smell. However, these improvements often go unnoticed until someone points them out. Sensitivity to odors increases a lot, which can be uncomfortable, especially in crowds.

Your taste buds also become more sensitive, and you might start tasting the water you drink. This sensitivity makes it important to choose distilled or alkaline water. Spring water or purified water might taste rough and feel scratchy in your throat. To manage oral health, brush your teeth without toothpaste and use distilled water. Mouthwash can help, but be very careful not to swallow it.

Phase three is often the time when you feel the most spiritual bliss. You become closer to the Lord, with a profound sense of peace and freedom filling you. Your emotional stability increases, and you become less affected by external events. Your confidence grows as insecurities fade, and materialistic and selfish desires diminish. Anxieties, fears, and self-image concerns start to break away and lose their power over you. If there are demonic strongholds in your life, you'll start to notice freedom. Emotions you've never experienced before may come to the surface as well.

Some days, you might feel a bit edgy or groggy, but this is part of the spiritual warfare occurring. Remember: fasting often reveals deeper emotional and spiritual issues. This phase helps clear away the clutter, which highlights underlying issues you may not have been aware of. You become more sensitive to the spiritual realm, which helps you to not be affected by physical distractions and stresses.

You can think of fasting like lying in a dark, cluttered room filled with boxes. Initially, in phase one, you're dormant and unaware of the clutter, and you have a blindfold on. By phase two, the blindfold comes off, and you start to feel around the dark room.

By phase three, a light turns on, revealing all of the clutter that needs to be addressed.

These boxes represent distractions, addictions, and strongholds in your life. Fasting helps you recognize and clear them out. For example, childhood wounds or lies you believed about yourself become apparent. The Holy Spirit will highlight these issues, allowing you to process and heal from them. As you clear the clutter, you may discover new spiritual insights, like a hidden closet where Jesus is waiting to be let in. You may discover new gifts and talents about yourself that were locked up in the closet.

You may find things you've been holding on to that need to be thrown away or people you need to forgive (including yourself). There may be certain relationships that you need to let go of or restore.

During this phase, you will also become more aware of the spiritual realm. You will feel closer to the Holy Spirit, sensing His presence more intensely than ever before. This makes you less bothered by worldly concerns and more focused on spiritual growth. For those not yet born again, this phase can be a time of significant spiritual revelation and encounter with Jesus.

To navigate this phase, spend a lot of time in prayer, reading the Bible, and worshiping the Lord. Learn to rest with Jesus, finding strength and clarity in His presence. Allow the Holy Spirit to address deep-seated issues, even those that are particularly painful or difficult to confront. Remember, the physical discomforts are all part of the fasting process, and pressing through them is key to gaining deeper spiritual breakthroughs.

Phase three is often transformative, both physically and spiritually. It's a time of profound detoxification, heightened senses, and spiritual clarity. As you clear the clutter from your life, you become more aligned with God's plan and more sensitive to the spiritual realm. This phase lays the groundwork for even deeper experiences and revelations in the final phase of your fast.

Powerful Prayer: "Holy Spirit, what work are you doing in my heart? What needs to be healed? What needs to change in my life?"

Phase Four: Days Twenty-One to Forty

Phase four of a prolonged fast, which generally covers days twenty-one through forty, is a difficult and slow period. Time seems to drag, and the days will tend to feel long and boring. Staying occupied can help the days pass more quickly and take your mind off the fast.

However, it's important not to fill your time with distractions just to keep busy. This phase is especially challenging because you're nearing the end, and the temptation to think about food grows stronger. In my experience, I've sometimes found myself looking at pictures of food or thinking about recipes I want to try after the fast. It takes discipline to avoid these distractions and stay focused. Fortunately, your mind becomes more stable during this time, which allows you to block out distractions and not let them affect you.

This phase is usually a spiritual battle. It's intense, and you might feel like quitting early because of it. Doubts about the purpose and effectiveness of the fast can creep in. The enemy might try to convince you that you're wasting your time. You might feel like you're not hearing from God, but He is still close. Learn to slow down and rest with God during this time so He can bring powerful and energizing moments that sustain you for the remaining days. Even when you feel good, it's important to rest and thank God for the strength He provides.

The enemy will try to make you quit, even using seemingly harmless thoughts like *You've come a long way; you can stop now.*

This is where discernment is so very important. Physically, hunger might return during this phase, but for most people, true hunger typically doesn't come back until around forty days or later. It's hard to describe what real hunger feels like, but it might be similar to the feeling of your stomach "eating itself" that you experienced at the beginning of the fast.

Another common sign is the tongue starting to clear up. The whitening residue fades away completely. Again, use discernment because sometimes this is not always the case when hunger returns. It may return when the tongue is still white, and your tongue could become clear even though hunger hasn't returned.

Unless you feel clearly led by God to fast for more than forty days, it's almost always best to follow Jesus's example and end the fast at forty days. Sometimes, natural hunger returns before the end of phase four, but this isn't always true hunger. For instance, on day thirty-eight of one of my fasts, I was looking at pictures of food, and my stomach started to growl. I drank water, which my stomach couldn't keep down, and I vomited. I mistakenly thought this was true hunger and ended the fast prematurely because of a lack of knowledge and panic about throwing up.

During this phase, you might experience nausea, difficulty drinking water, and increased weakness to the point where all you can do is lay in bed. It's important to stay hydrated, even if you don't feel like drinking water. Consistency is key, even if you start to dislike the taste of water.

You'll likely experience increased fatigue and decreased muscle strength. Some days, you might feel terrible because your body is still purging toxins that have accumulated over years of poor diet. It's important to remember that fasting isn't just about physical health; it's a spiritual journey seeking God's will, clearing out the clutter, and healing.

In this phase, your body is cleaning out dead tissues and healing both naturally and supernaturally. God designed our bodies to heal physically, mentally, emotionally, and spiritually. Ketone levels in your blood might spike during this phase of the fast, which can cause rashes or other skin issues. For example, I mentioned that I experienced a keto rash during my first prolonged fast, which scared me into breaking the fast prematurely. I later learned this is a normal part of the detox process. Such physical symptoms can vary and might include skin redness or fainting, but they shouldn't be reasons to panic and stop the fast.

These symptoms typically clear up after day thirty. The more you fast, the less severe these symptoms become as your body continues to heal. Though I panicked and ended my first long fast early, over time, as my faith and understanding grew, I learned to trust the Lord to heal me. This encouraged me to push through subsequent fasts, and I saw physical healing as a result.

Fasting is a time to grow in faith by relying on Jesus. You're seeking the Lord with a heart willing to surrender everything to Him. Maintaining this mentality will help you push through the difficult days. Trust that you are in God's hands, even if you feel weak or ill, and let Him reassure you.

By this stage of the fast, spiritual growth should be evident. This phase allows for profound inner healing that might not have been possible in earlier phases. As distractions and clutter in your life have begun to clear out, the Lord will identify and help remove some deep-seated issues, sometimes even generational wounds. You may start to notice cracks and flaws in your "spiritual room" that need fixing. Jesus will help you repair them.

New habits and spiritual disciplines often form during this phase. You might find yourself reading the Bible daily or spending more time in prayer, habits that can easily continue even after the fast ends. Gifts and fruit of the Holy Spirit begin to manifest and bring revelation. You'll understand the gifts and allow the Holy Spirit to operate through you. This phase strengthens your faith, making you spiritually stronger, similar to the way you can lift heavier weights after you've spent some time lifting lighter ones.

Since generational iniquities are deeply rooted, this is the phase where those roots are dug up and severed. For example, there may be a history of drinking in your family, abuse, sexual immorality, unbelief, religion, drugs, gluttony, manipulation, fear, anxiety, depression, or anger. Whatever the case in your personal life, this phase brings you head-on with these issues and allows Jesus to deal with them.

As a personal example, fasting removed my "fear of man," people-pleasing, and insecurities and improved my confidence about sharing my faith. There's an increased hunger to reach lost souls, no matter the cost. These are some examples of fruits that lasted well after the fast and have become vital in my life. These kinds of changes often manifest in your relationships and daily life as you establish new, positive behaviors that persist after the fast.

In the end, this final phase of your fast is a time of intense physical and spiritual cleansing. It will challenge you to rely deeply on God, which can lead to healing on many levels, a shattering of unbelief, an explosion of faith, freedom from bondage and demonic oppression, sensitivity to the Holy Spirit, and total reliance on Him. The habits and lessons learned during this phase are going to significantly transform your life and strengthen your faith.

Powerful Prayer: "Jesus, my life is in Your hands. Use me as You please. I yield my ways to You. Holy Spirit, what is my purpose on this earth? What are you speaking to me?"

The Four Phases of Fasting

Phase	Mental/ Emotional	Physical	Spiritual
Phase One Days 1–5	• temptation to quit • thoughts of food • realization of the stronghold of food, and weakness of the flesh • clearing of confusion	• intense withdrawal headaches • food cravings • feeling sick/tired • intense detoxification	• spiritual growth begins • need for focus • doubts and fear • unaware of unbelief • faith as tiny as a mustard seed
Phase Two Days 6–12	• dreams about food • doubts and frustration • internal self-reflection begins/grows • increased mental clarity	• hunger pangs decrease • weakness leaves the body	• prayer gives bursts of energy • seek Jesus for strength and comfort • faith of the mustard seed begins to sprout
Phase Three Days 13–20	• sharper focus • improved mental state • confidence grows • greater control of emotions • doubts come and go but not as often	• "cruise control" • hunger subsides • minor physical challenges • renewed strength • enhanced senses	• spiritual bliss • clearing away the clutter • closeness to the Holy Spirit • faith of the mustard seed has grown into a tall plant
Phase Four Days 21–40	• boredom • profound mental and emotional stability • developing new habits • wrestling with depression, loneliness, thoughts of quitting come and go	• nausea • weakness and fatigue • rashes and skin issues • physical cleansing • tongue starts to clear up • younger appearance • less body fat • more muscle tone	• spiritual warfare • surrendered to Jesus • profound spiritual growth • breaking generational curses • faith of the mustard seed is fully grown into a tree where others can come dwell and feed off of

Live More Fully

When you fast, you begin to experience life in a new, more spiritual way. Your understanding of the Bible deepens, and you gain a fresh perspective on the world around you. Your eyes are opened, and you develop a strong sense of discernment. This helps you understand God's plan for your life, make better decisions for your family and relationships, improve your work, and grow closer to Jesus.

In H. M. Shelton's book *The Science and Fine Art of Fasting*, the author talks about fasting being common among ancient Egyptians, who used it for secular purposes but gained wisdom and insights through it.[36] Moses fasted on Mount Sinai and came down with enlightenment, the Ten Commandments, and a profound encounter with God.

During a fast, you, too, are likely to experience revelations and encounters with the Lord, although these experiences will vary from person to person and fast to fast. Some people have dramatic encounters, like seeing Jesus in their room, while others might merely feel His presence in more subtle ways. The exciting part of fasting is this potential to encounter Jesus, feel His love, experience His power like never before, and allow Him to work in your heart. Fasting trains you to live more fully in the spiritual realm and to grow in your faith. Knowing that should help you hang in there through the difficult days.

CHAPTER 8: BREAKING THE FAST

In John chapter 21, there's a story that takes place after Jesus's resurrection. He appears to some of His disciples on the shores of the Sea of Galilee while they are out fishing. They've been fishing all night but haven't caught anything, so He tells them, "Throw your net on the right side of the boat, and you will find some."

They follow His advice, and sure enough, they catch so many fish that they can't even pull the net into the boat. They have to tow it back to shore. The disciples could be fasting at this moment. John 21:3 says they went out that night to fish but caught nothing. Therefore, they fished all night, and it could be that they didn't eat. However, importantly, when they arrive on land again, they find Jesus cooking breakfast. As it says in verse 9 in the English Standard Version, "When they got out on land, they saw a charcoal fire in place, with fish laid out on it, and bread."

In John 21:12, Jesus invites them to breakfast. This is the first time in the New Testament that the word "breakfast" is used. The word literally means "breaking a fast." The length isn't important here, but it is noteworthy that even short fasts have power. The point is that the disciples were on a fast and received revelation (they heard Jesus), got direction (they tossed the net on the other side), and their eyes opened (they saw it was Jesus). A fast draws you closer to Jesus.

When you finally break your fast, you should use that time to draw near to Jesus, just as the disciples did when they shared a meal with Him beside the Sea of Galilee. As you did during the fast, use this time to draw near and spend time with Him. It's important to continue the breaking of the fast with the intention of continuing to spend time with Jesus. The "heavy lifting" is done. The burden of the fast is no longer on you. This is a time to honor Jesus with each meal. Treat each meal as if Jesus was sitting next to you and partaking in the meal with you.

Sometimes, after a fast, the temptation is to go back to your old way of living. The disciples did just that once Jesus's earthly ministry was finished. They didn't know what to do, so they went back to fishing, but Jesus called them to spend time with Him and reminded them of their true calling and reason for living. Jesus wants to spend time with you at each meal.

Continue this new life, journey, and revelation you've received during the fast as you break and the days that follow beyond. Be attentive. Jesus is always speaking, giving direction, and revealing Himself to you.

Eating Too Much Too Soon

Your focus should be on Jesus, but you also have to be mindful of your physical condition. Once you have fasted for at least twenty-one days, you can't immediately return to your old eating habits or diet. This journey is going to change the way your body needs food so your body won't desire processed junk food. You also won't need to eat three meals a day with snacks in between.

When I finished my first fast, it was hard to resist eating too much too quickly. The hard part was knowing I could eat again but being patient about breaking the fast slowly. I focused on introducing food back into my system so I could get back to my old eating habits, and as a result, I began to eat more than I needed. There were many times I overate and forced myself to throw up because my stomach was in so much pain. My body wasn't yet ready to process those foods, and I paid a price for it. I share this so you don't make the same mistakes or fall into the trap of old eating habits.

Remember: It's important to break your fast slowly and pay attention to how your body reacts to each reintroduced food. My friend Andrea, who fasted for forty days, ate meat too quickly, and her ankles swelled up. She panicked, thinking she had ruined her fast. However, by going back to fasting for a couple of days, the swelling (water retention) subsided as her body adjusted to breaking the fast. Here's her testimony about the powerful journey of her forty-day fast:

> I went on a forty-day fast because of personal issues and a need to seek God's direction. I wasn't sure if I could sustain it for the full forty days, but it helped to understand that the physical reactions from not eating were temporary, and I didn't let them discourage me. In my weakened state, I found myself reflecting on what Jesus experienced during His fast, which drew me closer to God. Feeling weak led me to pray more, and I relied heavily on prayer throughout. A forty-day fast can't be done in your own strength—you must fully submit your mind and heart to Jesus and deny the distractions around you. Don't focus on food. Surrender completely to God, and He will sustain you during the fast. When breaking the fast, maintaining prayer was important. I still felt weak and wanted to eat everything, but I learned I couldn't return to my old eating habits. All my body needed was a small amount of nutrient-dense

food. This fast was the best thing I've ever done—it drew me closer to God.

And here is testimony on breaking a fast from Nick Thummel:

> Getting my body back to functioning with food has been a tremendous transition as well. I was cautious on food choices and slowly getting back into eating fruits and vegetables. Water started to taste good again. I did feel like I ate too many vegetables several days after the fast and felt like I was walking back into old food habits of overeating. I feel like the battle continues. Some of this is changing my thinking and aligning my habits with Jesus and not my fleshly desires. Those chapters have yet to be written in my book as I learn to navigate the breaking and journey of completing my first long fast. I do have concerns. I have four decades of history of overeating and that battle with the flesh. I'm continuing to pray for intimacy with Jesus. There's definitely a heightened awareness of my actions and failures and finding the root cause. I'm going to continue to walk with the Lord and let Him lead me.

Fortunately, a prolonged fast makes you more sensitive to your body. You can more easily tell when your body has received the desired nutrition, and most of the time, you won't feel full at that point. But it takes a lot of discipline because the typical American diet is full of rich foods, and we tend to think it is normal to eat until the body feels full. However, this is not actually healthy. By the time you feel full, you've taken in more than what your body needs.

If you find yourself overeating, eating too much too soon, eating too often, and you notice similar symptoms, just slow down and go back to fasting if need be. Your body will adjust. Take your time and eat slowly. Notice the smells and tastes of the food. Food is going to taste better, and you will find that fruits and vegetables are more enjoyable. Be thankful for the opportunity to eat. Just as Jesus gave food to His disciples, the food you eat after fasting is a blessing from Him. Treat it as such, and don't be in a hurry.

Bear in mind that you're supposed to wean yourself back into food over the same number of days that you fasted. In other words, if you fasted for seven days, you're supposed to take seven more days to gradually break the fast. During that time, you need to reintroduce food a little bit at a time and avoid meat altogether.

You need to wake up your digestive system slowly after it's been resting. Speaking more precisely, your intestines have tiny hairlike structures called villi that become dormant during fasting.[37] As you start eating again, they wake up slowly. If you eat heavy foods like meat too soon, it can damage your digestive system and cause health problems.

Here is a more precise timeline for breaking your fast in a way that will gradually wean you back onto food. I created this plan based on my experiences of breaking many long fasts through trial and error. Use this as a guide, and try to stick to the recommended eating times and meals. The important thing is to break slowly and listen to your body.

Breaking Your Fast Timeline

- Remember: Honor Jesus in the breaking of the fast.
- Breaking the fast is still part of the fast.
- Treat each meal as an appointed time, with Jesus sitting with you, eating.
- Breaking the fast will be more challenging than the fast itself.

- If you've had trouble with food in the past, get an accountability partner to help you break the fast.
- I've found that breaking with whole organic fruits and vegetables works best.
- Stay in a fasted state by only eating what your body needs; don't overeat or eat until you're full.
- Stick with this diet until you've completed the same number of days you've fasted (e.g., seven days of fasting, break the fast over seven days; twenty-one days, break for twenty-one days, etc.).
- Don't return to old eating habits:
  › Junk food (candy, sugar, chips, processed foods, dairy, meats, or a diet rich in seasonings, etc.).
  › Eating until you're full or your stomach hurts.
  › Eating when you don't feel the need to eat. (It's better to skip a meal if your body doesn't need food than to overnourish. Overnourishment leads to bodily malfunction and diseases.)
- Your body is still healing and cleansing from the fast. Eat whole, healthy foods that grow and are life-giving as your body begins to replenish and build up.
- Stay in tune with your body. You will notice once you've broken the fast, you likely won't need to eat three meals a day or snack. Most likely, your body will only need one meal full of life-giving food. I recommend eating this meal around dinnertime as it takes energy to digest food, and it will make you tired. Your body processes the food and repairs itself through the night while you sleep. When you wake up, you will feel refreshed, energized, and ready to go through your day with mental clarity.
- Your body will be brand new, operating optimally, and your energy levels will skyrocket.
- Remember: be patient!

Practice Guideline for Breaking a Fast of One to Forty Days

The following process for breaking a fast can be used for any length of fasting but is especially well suited for fasts of up to twenty-one days. If you fasted anywhere from one to ten days, feel free to start following the breaking guidelines from days three to five. For longer fasts, anywhere from ten to twenty-one days, I recommend adding a day or two of juicing before following the practical guidelines. For twenty-one to forty days, start with three to five days of juicing before following the practical guidelines. It's a good idea to break the fast with freshly squeezed organic juice and gradually transition from juice to whole fruit. The longer you can stay on juice, the better (a cold-press juicer is a great investment).

Tips

- You can eat the fruit of your choice, but the recommended types are listed.
- Mealtimes can vary based on when you break and start your first meal until you go to sleep, but the suggested times are recommended.
- Give your body a break from food when you sleep (from your last meal until the first meal the next day).
- Meal sizes are suggested (don't overeat or eat until full, and it's OK if you don't feel full).
- I encourage squeezing one to two days' worth of juice at a time and storing it in mason jars in the fridge.
- Drink as much water as you like throughout the day.

Day One

- 7:00 a.m. (or your first meal): 2–4 oz/one handful of watermelon or a whole organic Honeycrisp apple.
- 1:30 p.m. (or your second meal): 2–4 oz/one cluster/handful of organic red seedless grapes.
- 7:00 p.m. (or your third meal): 2–4 oz/one handful/one pint of organic blueberries.

Day Two

- 5:00 a.m.–7:00 a.m. (or your first meal): 4–6 oz. of fruit of your choice or one organic Honeycrisp apple.
- 9:00 a.m.–11:00 a.m.: 4–6 oz. of fruit of your choice or one cluster of organic red seedless grapes.
- 12:00 p.m.–2:00 p.m. Optional in-between meal drink: 4–6 oz. of freshly squeezed organic lemon juice, diluted with 8 oz. of water, and added vitamin B12, probiotic, and a multivitamin of your choice.
- 3:00 p.m.: 4–6 oz. of fruit of your choice.
- 6:00 p.m.–8:00 p.m.: 4–6 oz. of fruit of your choice or organic blueberries.

Days Three to Five

- 5:00 a.m.–7:00 a.m. (or your first meal): 6–8 oz. of fruit of your choice or a whole organic Honeycrisp apple.
- 10:00 a.m.–12:00 p.m.: 8–10 oz. of fruit of your choice.

- Optional in-between meal drink: 4–6 oz. of freshly squeezed organic lemon juice, diluted with 8 oz. of water, and added vitamin B12, probiotic, and a multivitamin of your choice.
- 4:00 p.m.–6:00 p.m.: 10 oz. of fruit of your choice or a whole Honeycrisp apple.
- 8:00 p.m.–10:00 p.m. (or final meal before bed): 10–12 oz. of fruit of your choice or whole Honeycrisp apples.

Days Six to Ten

- You can start incorporating vegetable soup or cooked veggies for dinner/final meal before bed.
- Stay away from adding oil or seasonings to your vegetables.
- Around this time of breaking the fast, temptations may creep in to break your fast too quickly or give in to cravings/old eating habits.
- 5:00 a.m.–7:00 a.m. (or your first meal): 12–16 oz. of fruit of your choice or Honeycrisp apples.
- Pay attention to your body—if you feel you're not satiated, it's OK to adjust the amount of fruit.
- 10:00 a.m.–12:00 p.m.: 12–16 oz. of fruit of your choice.
- Optional in-between meal drink: 4–6 oz. of freshly squeezed organic lemon juice, diluted with 8 oz. of water, and added vitamin B12, probiotic, and a multivitamin of your choice.
- 5:00 p.m.–7:00 p.m. (or your final meal): Vegetable soup, or air-fried/baked vegetables of your choice.
- This meal size may vary but can be larger than your typical meals up until this point.
- Don't overeat; eat until satiated. Listen to your body and give it what it needs.

Days Eleven to Sixteen

- You can start incorporating salads for lunch.
- You can start incorporating small amounts of potatoes, rice, quinoa, or starchier foods for dinner.
- 5:00 a.m.–7:00 a.m. (or your first meal): Your choice of fruit until your body feels satiated. Don't overeat. It is recommended to stick to one type of fruit per meal.
- 10:00 a.m.–12:00 p.m. (or lunchtime): Your choice of fruit or salad until your body feels satiated.
- Keep salads simple with a mix of vegetables, and avoid dressings.
- Optional in-between meal drink: 4–6 oz. of freshly squeezed organic lemon juice, diluted with 8 oz. of water, and added vitamin B12, probiotic, and a multivitamin of your choice.
- 5:00 p.m.–7:00 p.m. (dinner or your final meal before bed): Vegetable soup with added potatoes, rice, beans, or quinoa, or a bowl of air-fried vegetables (onions, garlic, broccoli, mixed peppers, sweet potatoes, carrots, cauliflower, mushrooms) with added starchier foods.

Days Seventeen to Twenty-One

- Squeeze one lemon into a large jug of water (1–3 liters) and drink throughout the day.
- Notice that the starchier or heavier the meal is at dinner, or when new foods are reintroduced, the more time it takes to digest. You may not feel the need to eat a morning meal.
- 5:00 a.m.–7:00 a.m. (optional first meal—don't eat if you don't feel hungry or the need): Juice, fruit, or rest are always recommended for the first mealtime.

- It may be best to simply have the optional in-between meal drink: 4–6 oz. of freshly squeezed organic lemon juice, diluted with 8 oz. of water, and added vitamin B12, probiotic, and a multivitamin of your choice.
- 10:00 a.m.–12:00 p.m.: Your choice of food: fruits or salads.
- Keep the meals as fresh as possible with no added seasonings, dressings, or oils.
- 5:00 p.m.–7:00 p.m.: I personally recommend staying on fruits and vegetables as part of your daily diet.
- This is a good time to add whole organic nuts without seasoning to your diet.
- If you don't mind using dairy, you can use this mealtime to introduce small amounts of new foods like eggs, oatmeal, bread, milk, vegan protein shakes, different vegetables, and minimally processed pasta.
- New foods introduced should range from 2–4 oz. and can be gradually increased by 2 oz. at the next dinner meal.

Days Twenty-Two to Forty

- At this point, when breaking the fast, stay consistent with your diet.
- Don't snack between meals.
- Don't go back to processed foods.
- Stay off meat for as long as you can (I recommend not eating meat or dairy anymore).
- If you do go back to eating meat, try to wait until you've completely finished forty days of breaking the fast before introducing small amounts at dinner.

Practice Guideline for Breaking a Fast of Twenty-One to Forty Days

This guideline offers a slight adjustment intended to help you break a fast of twenty-one to forty days. The major differences occur during the first three to five days of breaking the fast and easing into solid food.

The First One to Five Days

- 6–8 oz. of freshly squeezed organic juice (recommended: apple, grape, cherry, spinach, carrots, cucumber, grapefruit) diluted with an equal amount of water (6–8 oz) for a total of 12–16 oz.
- Mixing in sauerkraut or pickle juice for one of the meals will help with lightheadedness, digestion, and getting a little sodium back into your body.
- You can increase the amount of juice by 2 oz. each day or as your body needs (it's best to limit your juice intake to 16 oz. per meal).
- You can continue to dilute the juice with equal amounts of water or simply increase the juice amount without increasing the water. (Example: 8 oz. of juice + 6 oz. of water. The next day, 10 oz. of juice + 6 oz. of water, etc.).
- Juice one kind of fruit and don't mix fruits. You can drink different fruit juices for each mealtime (e.g., one mealtime can be apple juice, another grape juice).
- Vegetable juices like spinach can be mixed with other juicier green vegetables.
- Drink every 2–3 hours or as your body needs within a 12–14 hour time frame. (Example: If you start at 6:00 a.m., your last juice meal should be around 6:00–8:00 p.m. before you go to sleep).

- Give your body a break during sleep.

Day Six

- Begin to replace your last juice meal with solid fruit.
- The reason to replace the final meal with whole fruit is because it's solid and heavier, requiring more energy and time to digest, which can make you more tired and allow for better sleep.
- 7:00 a.m. (or your first meal): Drink freshly squeezed juice of your choice (it's OK to start mixing juices at this point).
- Limit your juice amount to 16 oz.
- You can add additional water to the 16 oz. of juice to dilute it to your liking.
- Next meals: all juice, every 2–3 hours, until the final meal before bed.
- 7:00–9:00 p.m. (or your final meal before bed): Eat one type of whole fruit (listen to your body and don't overeat or eat until you're full).

Day Seven

- Replace the last two juice meals with whole fruit.
- Remember to allow more time between whole fruit meals (average 4–5 hours between meals).
- 7:00 a.m. (or your first meal): Drink freshly squeezed juice of your choice.
- Next meals: all juice, every 2–3 hours, until your final two mealtimes (listen to your body).

- 4:00–5:00 p.m. (or second-to-last meal): Eat one type of whole fruit (listen to your body and don't overeat or eat until you're full).
- Allow 4–5 hours until your next mealtime.
- 8:00–9:00 p.m. (or final meal before bed): Eat one type of whole fruit (listen to your body and don't overeat or eat until you're full).

Day Eight

- Start your day with juice, and replace the rest of your juice meals with whole fruit throughout the day.
- Remember to allow more time between whole fruit meals (average 4–5 hours between meals).
- 7:00 a.m. (or your first meal): Drink freshly squeezed juice of your choice.
- 9:00–10:00 a.m. (or next meal): Drink freshly squeezed juice of your choice.
- 11:00 a.m.–12:00 p.m. (or next meal): Eat one type of whole fruit (listen to your body and don't overeat or eat until you're full).
- 4:00–5:00 p.m. (or your next meal): Eat one type of whole fruit (listen to your body and don't overeat or eat until you're full).
- 8:00–9:00 p.m. (or your final meal before bed): Eat one type of whole fruit (listen to your body and don't overeat or eat until you're full).

Day Nine-Plus

- You can start following the one- to twenty-one-day breaking-of-the-fast plan above.

- Gradually increase your fruit intake for each meal, one day at a time.
- The larger the meal, the more time you should allow between meals to let your body digest.

Additionally, the below alternative "refeeding" schedule was recommended by Loren Lockman, wellness advocate, fasting expert, and founder of the Tanglewood Wellness Center.[38]

Loren Lockman's Breaking/Refeeding Schedule

- Day One: 2 oz. of watermelon or papaya every two hours from 10:00 a.m. to 6:00 p.m. Choose one fruit for the whole day.
- Day Two: 4 oz. of watermelon every 2.5 hours from 9:00 a.m. to 7:00 p.m.
- Day Three: Depending on how you did on day two, eat between 6 and 8 oz. of watermelon, papaya, cantaloupe, or other melon every three hours from 9:00 a.m. to 6:00 p.m.
- Days Four to Seven: Increase quantity by about 4 oz. each day, eating four times between 9:00 a.m. and 6:00 p.m. (every three hours). You can add one acidic fruit meal per day starting on day four if you feel up to it.
- Days Eight and Beyond: Whole, ripe organic fruits and simple green salads. Nothing dehydrated, and very little fat.

Lockman's Note: You may want to substitute other fruits if you can't get watermelon or papaya. In fact, if you're not in a warm climate, I wouldn't necessarily recommend watermelon [unless you get it when it's in season]. You can use apples, pears, or other juicy fruits as well. The goal is to very slowly increase your food intake to jump-start your appetite and encourage your metabolism to stay as low as possible, making your system as efficient as you can.

When you begin to eat, stop drinking thirty minutes before each meal and wait forty-five minutes after eating to drink again. This means there will be only about a thirty-minute window to drink on the first day, so you'll need to spend your day drinking, eating, and resting in between. By around the third day, you might be ready for some very light exercise, increasing it slowly each day thereafter. Be careful not to overdo it too quickly—there's no rush, and you don't want to set yourself back.

Interestingly, Loren doesn't recommend juicing because nutrients and fiber are lost. In his estimation, juicing only spikes sugar levels and doesn't aid in the cleansing process. Whole fruits are recommended because they retain all the nutrients, and fiber is key. The water from the fruit is also very important, as it rehydrates the body and provides 70 to 80 percent of the water needed for the cells, helping to continue cleansing the system. His breaking method can be used for fasts ranging one to forty days.

Personally, I've found juicing helps the body absorb nutrients more quickly and prevents overeating or taking in too much food too quickly at the beginning of breaking the fast. I've added his perspective so that you can try both methods if you'd like and see which works best for you.

Above All

Above all, your real focus should be on the *spiritual* fruits of the fast, which we will talk about in the next chapter. Don't become obsessed with food again as soon as the fast is over. Instead, spend plenty of time staying close to the Lord, trusting Him, and listening to Him.

In Genesis 15, we are told that Abraham (then called Abram) was afraid of what would become of his family. He had no son, so a servant was poised to inherit his estate. But God spoke to Abraham, made a covenant with him, and revealed His plans for him. He promised that Abraham would have a son and, more than that, he would have as many descendants as there were stars in the sky. We are told in verse 6, "Abram believed the Lord, and he credited it to him as righteousness." In other words, God had a plan for his life, and He just wanted Abraham to trust Him.

That's what God asks of all of us: "Trust that I have a plan for you" (Jeremiah 29:11, paraphrase).

Similarly, when you fast, it's important to remember that God *already* has a plan for your life. Often, we try to force things to happen by our own efforts, but God's purpose is already laid out for us. We just need to rest and trust in Him.

So take your time breaking the fast. Rest. Stay close to the Lord. Listen to Him and trust Him. Don't get in a rush. He may use this time to confirm and clarify some things you experienced during the fast. It can be helpful to have a friend supporting you through the breaking process for the sake of accountability and safety.

Just be mindful as you reintroduce food to maintain self-control. It's common to overeat or eat things your body isn't ready for, especially as more freedom with food is regained. On average, you'll put back a pound every day. Don't stress about being too skinny or gaining weight too quickly. As I said, instead of eating until you feel stuffed, listen carefully to your body and stop when you've had enough. As you properly break the fast by following these guidelines, your weight will naturally level out. Your body will get to its natural weight.

During the fast, you've spent time diving into the Bible and praying. As you come out of the fast, continue these practices. You may find that you have a deeper understanding of the Scriptures and a stronger connection to God now.

Above all, breaking a fast requires patience, self-control, and a commitment to spiritual growth. Stay consistent with your prayer and Bible-reading habits, and avoid returning to old, unhealthy habits like excessive TV or social media use. Instead, keep focusing on seeking the Lord and feeding your spirit. He is not done working in you!

CHAPTER 9: FRUITS OF THE FAST

Fasting is a powerful and transformative practice with profound effects on the physical, spiritual, mental, and emotional aspects of life. Imagine a tree that bears different types of fruit—apples, pears, oranges, or plums. In one season, it may produce a certain fruit, and in another, something entirely different. Some fruits appear quickly, while others take time to mature. Though it's hard to predict the exact "fruit" you'll experience from fasting, you can be certain it will be life-changing.

What are some of these "fruits" in practical terms? Fasting discovers and deepens your spiritual gifts, enhancing your understanding of the gifts of the Holy Spirit and using them while operating out of love, not selfish gain. It reveals your true self, the state of your brokenness because of sin, fosters inner healing, and brings clarity to your sense of purpose. Through fasting, you embark on a journey of growth that touches every part of your life.

Spiritual Growth

Spiritual encounters, growth, and restoration often accompany fasting. The spiritual benefits are abundant, and the reason is clear: Fasting allows you to surrender your desires and align with God's will, creating space for transformative experiences. No matter where you are in your spiritual journey, fasting offers an opportunity to encounter Jesus, feel His love, and surrender to Him more fully.

This surrender aligns your prayers with God's intentions. Through self-denial, your desires shift from personal gain—like wealth or possessions—to deeper values such as love, peace, and a desire to serve others.

Fasting also enables you to bless others, becoming a vessel for the Holy Spirit's power. God can work through you to uplift and support those in need, break chains of sin, release generational burdens, and deepen the impact of prayer. As you fast, your faith grows stronger, empowering you to believe in the impossible. Indeed, fasting is one of the most powerful ways to build faith and strengthen your spiritual "muscle memory" in a way few other practices can.

Led by the Holy Spirit

When you're fasting, you're stepping into God's plan in the spiritual realm, preparing yourself to live out that plan as you conclude the fast. It's like following a path that's already been set before you. In fact, as you break the fast, you often feel a deeper connection to the Lord, with clarity and guidance from the Holy Spirit rather than your own desires. The flesh is subdued, which allows the Spirit to lead—how we are called to live continually. Galatians 5:25 reminds us that we should follow the Spirit's guidance in all we do.

After fasting, as you follow the Holy Spirit more closely, you may notice things coming together in unexpected ways. Small details may align, like finding a parking spot right when you need it or encountering someone whose words feel like confirmation from God. Opportunities may arise, doors may open or close, and God will meet your material needs while giving you vision and clarity for your next steps. If you've strayed from the path, the Spirit will gently realign you. These "coincidences" are, in fact, divine appointments that come when following the Spirit closely. Things often overlooked in life become clear: The Holy Spirit is working in every detail.

After prolonged consecrated fasts, I experienced sensitivity to the Holy Spirit's leading often. Many times, as I go about my day, I'm aware of the Holy Spirit highlighting someone at a grocery store. I get a prompting in my heart to go talk to the person and offer to pray for them. The person was going through something in that moment in their life where they were asking God for a sign. Here I am, being led by the Holy Spirit to talk to the person who ends up giving their life to Jesus.

Another story that comes to mind: There was a time after fasting when the Holy Spirit gave me a vision of a flower shop and told me to go to the nearest flower shop and bring the person working there a Bible. I obeyed the prompting in my heart. When I got there and told the people working there that I felt like I was supposed to give them a Bible, the flower shop owner responded, "I follow Jesus, but my son has been studying different religions and has been seeking God. He wants to learn more about the Bible." I never heard from the guy, but I know I was obedient to the Holy Spirit, and I have faith that the Bible will impact that family.

The fast gave me boldness and confidence through the Spirit's guidance. I often experience these encounters where the person decided to follow Jesus that day, or they've been looking for a sign for God to speak to them—showing me the power of fasting and God's ability to work through anyone open to His leading. I didn't force speaking engagements or promote myself; instead, I learned to wait, trusting that God would open the right doors in His timing.

Scripture offers a similar example in Acts 13. The church at Antioch was worshiping and fasting when the Holy Spirit said, "Set apart for me Barnabas and Saul for the work to which I have called them." Though Jesus had already purposed for them to spread the gospel, this plan was revealed to the church through prayer and fasting. The church, Paul, and Barnabas did not act by their own wisdom or force; instead, fasting aligned them with God's purpose. This fast demonstrated their expectancy and openness to the Lord's leading, allowing them to step into God's plan fully.

The exact number of days the early church spent worshiping and fasting isn't specified, but during that time, the Holy Spirit commanded them to set apart Saul (Paul) and Barnabas. This led to Antioch becoming the first Christian church to send missionaries to foreign nations.

Through fasting, they received a clear revelation of their mission. Fasting also heightened their sensitivity to the Holy Spirit, guiding them through each step and filling in the details of the mission. By aligning themselves with God's plan spiritually, they were able to follow it in the physical realm.

This story illustrates the type of "fruit" that fasting and prayer can bring. You may receive a revelation about your purpose, specific guidance for certain steps, or a larger vision for your life. Sometimes, the Holy Spirit may only reveal part of the picture or encourage you to wait patiently, trusting in divine timing.

This heightened sensitivity to the Holy Spirit helps keep you on the right path and strengthens your faith. Many try to navigate life by their own intellect, but without seeking guidance from God, this can lead to hardship, discord, confusion, and unintended consequences. Abraham's story provides a strong example.

In Genesis 15, God promises Abraham that his descendants will be as numerous as the stars. Abraham believes, but he's not given a time frame. By Genesis 16, about ten years have passed, and he and his wife, Sarai, are still without children. Sarai, reasoning in her own mind, believes God is preventing her from having a child. She suggests that Abraham marry Hagar, their Egyptian servant, to fulfill the promise through her. Instead of waiting on God, Abraham acts on Sarai's advice, taking matters into his own hands and having a child, Ishmael, with Hagar.

The immediate consequences are discord, resentment, and bitterness. In time, Hagar and Ishmael are sent away, which leads to lasting tensions between Ishmael's descendants and Isaac's—a conflict that persists to this day. Isaac was the son God had promised, but Abraham's impatience led him to act prematurely, trying to fulfill God's plan on his own terms.

How often have you tried to force God's plan because you couldn't wait or started to doubt? When you take steps without divine confirmation, it can lead to suffering and consequences. Fasting helps overcome these temptations, dispels doubt, and strengthens faith, enabling you to wait on God's timing and align with His will rather than your own.

You learn to yield to the Holy Spirit, who never forces Himself upon you but guides with gentleness, patience, kindness, and love. He may nudge you to act, speak, or simply wait quietly. Breaking a fast often reveals the fruit of this yielding, as the freedom to eat again brings new temptations. In those moments, the Holy Spirit may gently remind you, "You don't need that food; it's not good for your body." This can be the most challenging part of fasting, yet each time you choose to control your eating and make mindful choices, you strengthen your ability to follow the Spirit's guidance over your impulses, even in small details. This might mean holding back from speaking until the Spirit prompts you or waiting patiently instead of rushing ahead.

Building Perseverance

Now more than ever, people need to rediscover the process of persever-ance. In developed countries like the United States, people have grown accustomed to canceling, quitting, or walking away from challenging situations. When marriage becomes difficult, many choose divorce. If athletes are dissatisfied with a coach, team, or salary, they may quit or transfer. When a church member feels a pastor isn't moving quickly enough to support their idea, they find another congregation. Even missing a meal can leave someone irritable for the rest of the day.

With on-demand entertainment and instant access to almost every-thing, society has built a culture of instant gratification. As a result, when faced with trials or setbacks, many struggle with patience, problem-solving, and character-building. This erosion of character affects families, communities, and societies from the inside out.

"Blessed is the man who remains steadfast under trial, for when he has stood the test he will receive the crown of life, which God has promised to those who love him" (James 1:12). Life is full of trials. There will be times of trouble, unexpected circumstances, and hard-ship. Fasting teaches you to push through these moments, helping you develop perseverance and the ability to withstand challenges. Every time you resist the temptation to break a fast, you're building up your resilience.

This is similar to the journey of following Jesus. There will be per-secution, times when you want to give up, and moments when you can't have what you want. Fasting trains you to wait and persevere, cultivating character as described in Romans 5:3–4. When you're on day twenty of a forty-day fast and long for it to be over, you're learning to wait and endure the remaining days. This patience equips you for the trials in life, teaching you the strength to endure because you've practiced perseverance through fasting.

Proper Appetite

Fasting helps you confront and overcome food addictions and un-healthy eating habits. Many people unknowingly eat out of routine rather than necessity. If this resonates with you, fasting can break these habits and reveal that you don't need as much food as society often suggests. Since fasting brings you closer to Jesus and immerses you in the Holy Spirit, it reshapes your relationship with food, even as it deepens your spiritual connection with God.

A prolonged fast—lasting twenty-one to forty days—often brings a greater revelation of how much we tend to eat unnecessarily. You may realize that you don't need as much food as you once thought. Eating less can bring a newfound sense of contentment, peace, and joy.

As you fast, your spiritual appetite grows, replacing natural hunger with a desire for the Holy Spirit. This shift helps you move from being controlled by physical cravings to being led by the Spirit.

Becoming More Like Jesus

Fasting also helps heal broken parts of your soul, which leads to greater sanctification.

Sanctification is "the ongoing supernatural work of God to rescue justified sinners from the disease of sin and to conform them to the image of His Son: holy, Christlike, and empowered to do good works."[39] When a person places their faith in Jesus as Savior and surrenders their life to Him as Lord (Romans 10:9–10; Ephesians 1:13–14), they receive the gift of the Holy Spirit, who begins working within them, convicting them of sin. This spiritual growth shapes us to become more like Jesus (Philippians 1:6).

Before surrendering to Jesus, you might curse, lie, or be unaware of certain sin without much concern or conviction of sinning. But after choosing to follow Him, the Holy Spirit will begin to convict you each time you curse, lie, or sin, gradually renewing your heart and mind (Romans 8:6, 12:1–2). Over time, these behaviors lose their appeal, replaced by a desire to live in alignment with Christ.

Fasting deepens this process, increasing awareness of sin and sensitivity to the Holy Spirit's conviction. You realize that sin disrupts your peace and pushes away the Holy Spirit's presence. Through fasting, you come to cherish the closeness with the Spirit more than any worldly pleasure, which leads to greater obedience and intimacy with God.

As you grow more Christlike, others begin to see Jesus in you. This witness draws others to Him, leading to new believers and a multiplying effect of discipleship.

Physical, Mental, Emotional Healing

Fasting creates a dynamic opportunity for God to intervene and heal. Remarkably, God also designed the body to heal itself through fasting so that both physical and spiritual healing can take place. Physically, fasting is one of the most effective ways to support the body's natural healing process. It purifies the bloodstream, clears toxins, and allows the body to operate optimally. Common ailments like skin issues, indigestion, colds, and irregular body functions may improve or even resolve through fasting. Long-standing toxins or tumors may be reduced over time as the immune system strengthens. Fasting also promotes weight balance, helping the body reach its optimal, natural weight.

After a forty-day fast, many experience transformative mental and emotional improvements. By phase two or three of a prolonged fast (typically around days twelve to twenty-one), benefits often include enhanced eyesight, sharper hearing, and overall improved cognitive function. You may feel stronger, more energized, and spiritually attuned, with a clearer mind free from worry and distraction. Fasting sharpens focus, concentration, and the ability to absorb information, making learning and memory retention easier. Mentally, your mind can become more efficient, like a "supercomputer" for processing information.

Emotionally, fasting fosters patience, calmness, and mental clarity. Stress fades, which enables you to process emotions more effectively and identify the root of emotional issues. For example, it helps tremendously with grieving or in times of distress. Notice in these times, the body doesn't want to eat. Losing a loved one, divorce, breakups, moving, going through a transition, or a traumatic moment—when these happen in life, the natural appetite and desire for food goes away. The body instinctively needs to process those deep emotional feelings. In addition, there's a supernatural aspect where the Holy Spirit draws close to those who grieve. He is the Healer, Comforter, and Helper (John 14:26; 2 Corinthians 1:3–4). Fasting helps with processing heavy emotions and get through that process quicker.

Here is a testimony from my friend Petru Amarei:

> When I was invited to participate in a forty-day fast with the group led by Louis Trinca-Pasat at the beginning of 2023, I knew immediately I needed wisdom and guidance from the Lord. I had never practiced water fasting before. I was practicing the Daniel "fasts" regularly, but fasting for forty days was a huge challenge. The voices in my head were telling me, *Don't do it! You won't make it; you're on medication; you're going to die.*
>
> The mental, emotional, and spiritual battle began. I informed my family and asked God to help me decide. I was told to commit to seven days. As a confirmation (validation) that it was God speaking,

my wife also joined. It was an amazing and, at the same time, challenging experience. The first three days were very hard for me, and I almost gave up, but the Holy Spirit helped me to continue to complete the seven days as planned.

This experience helped me get out of my comfort zone and walk much closer to God. I also lost ten pounds and felt stronger physically, mentally, emotionally, and spiritually. At the beginning of 2024, I repeated the fast for ten days. To God be the glory!

Demonic Strongholds Broken

"For though we walk in the flesh, we are not waging war according to the flesh. For the weapons of our warfare are not of the flesh but have divine power to destroy strongholds. We destroy arguments and every lofty opinion raised against the knowledge of God and take every thought captive to obey Christ, being ready to punish every disobedience, when your obedience is complete" (2 Corinthians 10:3–6).

If you're struggling with habitual sin, it may be a sign of spiritual oppression. When the demonic influences a person through sin, generational iniquities, inner wounds, or lies they've embraced, fasting can be a path to freedom. A stronghold is something we turn to in order to numb the pain within our hearts, or something learned from a young age that has become a mindset. It may either result from demonic oppression or open the door to it. What does this mean practically?

Many turn to various things to avoid facing heart issues—jobs, relationships, sex, porn, drugs, idols, religion, and, subtly, food. Emotional barriers like people-pleasing, fear, greed, pride, isolation, anger, and insecurity are a few examples of walls people put up to protect their wounded hearts, running to anything other than Jesus. Most people are unaware of their strongholds or oppression until they experience a long fast.

One of the fruits of fasting is breaking free from strongholds that some call "habits," like drinking, smoking, and drug use, which can often be broken within three to five days of fasting. Freedom from deeper strongholds may require more prolonged, consecrated fasts of twenty-one to forty days, where you can find healing, revelation, and fulfillment in Jesus's love. Strongholds shatter, and though multiple fasts may be necessary, freedom is attainable.

If you've tried everything else to find freedom and healing without success, consider seeking Jesus in a forty-day fast and witness the transformation He can bring.

Breaking Generational Iniquities

Fasting fosters a deeper connection with the Holy Spirit and helps shift your focus from earthly desires to spiritual growth. As you cleanse your body and mind, you open yourself more fully to the Holy Spirit's presence, allowing Him to guide every aspect of your life. This transformation brings a renewed sense of purpose that empowers you to live according to God's plan and break free from generational iniquities.

Generational iniquities are patterns of sin that affect a family over many years due to either learned behaviors or spiritual influences. For example, in Genesis 13, Abraham lies in Egypt, claiming that his wife, Sarah, is his sister out of fear that Pharaoh might kill him to take her. This lie causes complications when Pharaoh, believing Sarah is unmarried, takes her into his household. Displeased, God sends a plague as punishment, and Abraham ultimately confesses, leading to their departure from Egypt.

Abraham repeats this behavior in Genesis 20, lying again to King Abimelech for similar reasons. The pattern continues into the next generation; in Genesis 26, Abraham's son Isaac, who wasn't even born during the earlier events, lies to King Abimelech, claiming his wife, Rebekah, is his sister. Isaac's behavior mirrors Abraham's, perpetuating a sinful pattern across generations.

This illustrates a generational iniquity—a destructive behavior that takes root in a family and continues from generation to generation. These patterns aren't always sinful behaviors; sometimes, they are emotional or relational habits. In my own family, for instance, a lack of affection persisted across generations. Growing up, I rarely expressed love or affection outwardly, a result of my parents' upbringing in a culture where openly showing emotions was not common. I wasn't fully aware of this generational pattern until I began long consecrated fasts.

When I recognized this emotional coldness in my own behavior, I knew it was something I wanted to change. I started by forgiving my parents for any past hurts, and I began to hug them and tell them I loved them. I began to talk about my feelings and emotions. I acknowledged the existence of my feelings and began to verbalize them. At first, it felt awkward, but I knew the Holy Spirit was guiding me. Through fasting, the Spirit empowered me to break this pattern and embrace a new way of relating to my family.

By breaking this cycle, I believe I broke a generational pattern. While this change may seem small, it was significant for me and my family. This is one example of how fasting can bring about positive changes, even in ways that might seem minor to others.

New Wineskin

In Mark 2:20–22 and Luke 5:37–39, Jesus is approached by John's disciples and the Pharisees, who frequently fasted out of religious duty.

According to Mosaic law, Jews were required to fast only once a year on the Day of Atonement. However, the Pharisees had added their own religious rules, including the practice of fasting twice a week. One day, they asked Jesus why He and His disciples didn't fast like them. Jesus responded, "The days will come when the bridegroom is taken away from them, and then they will fast in that day. No one sews a piece of unshrunk cloth on an old garment...And no one puts new wine into old wineskins." (Mark 2:20–22).

The twin parables teach that the old (Judaism) and the new (Christianity) are incompatible. Judaism is represented by the old garment and wineskin, while Christianity is the new garment and wineskin, filled with new wine.[40] Jesus would soon be crucified, rise from the grave, and ascend into heaven. Now is the time to fast, not from religious duty, but as a response to His love.

This passage specifically speaks of new life in Jesus. Those who surrender their lives to Him don't return to old practices or rules; they receive the Holy Spirit and become a new creation—new wineskins. "Therefore, if anyone is in Christ, he is a new creation. The old has passed away; behold, the new has come" (2 Corinthians 5:17). Fasting is no longer about religious duty on a certain day or following a strict fasting schedule. New life in the Holy Spirit will stir a spiritual hunger in you that will lead you to want to fast out of love. It becomes a response, a need, a desire, because the Holy Spirit hungers for the things of Jesus.

In the context of fasting, prolonged consecrated fasts of twenty-one to forty days expand your spiritual capacity. As a new wineskin, you allow your new nature to grow, enabling God to pour "new wine" into you. This means God can increase your understanding of the Bible, strengthen your faith, empower your prayer life, and refresh your desire for Jesus. You develop a deeper understanding that life is not about fulfilling personal desires but aligning with God's will and purposes. These long fasts strengthen you spiritually, preparing you to handle whatever God has in store.

Fasting also transforms you so that going back to old ways of self-centeredness or sin would be damaging. Fasting keeps your spiritual capacity fresh, opening doors for God to pour more into you. Through fasting, you become a new wineskin and invite God to fill you with new wine—His wisdom, guidance, and strength. God doesn't let new wineskins go unused; He pours into them and uses them in ways that lead to growth beyond what you might imagine.

Practical Ways God Answers

Fasting has led to many answered prayers in my life, and the experiences I've shared in this chapter are examples of its impact. Once, while in seminary, I really needed my own apartment—a quiet place to spend time with God. At the time, I had a roommate, which made it difficult. During a fast, I met someone looking for a roommate to save money, and we were able to swap apartments. That night, I prayed, asking God to provide for the increased rent. The next morning, I received a notification about a small crypto investment I'd made the year before, which had suddenly spiked in value. The profit was enough to cover the higher rent for the year and most of my meals—a clear answer to prayer and a testament to God's provision after fasting.

Fasting also brought clarity to my relationships. I realized I had been seeking relationships out of loneliness rather than a genuine desire to love and serve another person. Through fasting, God revealed deeper truths about His love and purpose, helping me avoid significant relationship mistakes. Rather than entering relationships from selfish motives, fasting exposed my intentions and showed me that the type of person I was pursuing wasn't aligned with God's calling for my life. Fasting aligns you with God's plan, and if marriage is part of that plan, fasting can bring clarity and confirmation about a potential spouse.

In addition to clarity, fasting has multiplied opportunities for ministry and increased spiritual anointing. After a twenty-one-day fast, I was invited to speak to high school athletes about my faith, a breakthrough that helped me overcome my fear of public speaking and share the gospel confidently. In December 2022, I undertook a twenty-four-day fast while praying about writing a book. Although it took some time to begin (the book you're now reading), the fast allowed me to surrender to God's timing.

Leading a fasting group has also taught me about growth, deliverance, and inner healing. Through fasting, I learned to listen to the Holy Spirit and address areas in my life that needed healing, even from childhood. It allowed me to confront painful memories and lies and, with God's help, overcome them. During a twenty-one-day fast in Providence, Rhode Island, I witnessed a man delivered from demonic oppression—a moment that opened my eyes to the power of deliverance ministry. I realized that fasting had prepared me for spiritual warfare by aligning my heart with God's will. I came to understand that, as a follower of Jesus, I have the authority to lead others in prayers for inner healing and deliverance.

On a trip to New Brunswick, Canada, I had the opportunity to put what I'd learned into practice. After studying the Bible and books on deliverance, I found myself helping people walk through inner healing and freedom from spiritual oppression. I witnessed many find peace and healing, letting God use me in ways I hadn't anticipated.

Since my first journey of a prolonged consecrated fast in May of 2020, I went from a person who sat in a chair at church and who knew *of* Jesus to *knowing* Jesus and traveling the world and telling people about the good news of Jesus all within a two-year span that continues to this day. In October 2023, Jesus would bring me back to the Philippines, the very same place I fully surrendered my life to

Jesus in 2020, this time not as a person seeking identity and purpose but to share the gospel and train people from other countries to do the same. Following Jesus and walking in obedience is a daily battle, but fasting has created these wells of spiritual living water. Whenever I'm thirsty, I can go back to them, take a drink, and be refreshed to keep running the race before me.

Through fasting, you will experience answered prayers and unexpected blessings. Some blessings may seem small, like an increase in joy or peace, while others may be larger, as God works in ways you never imagined. These answers to prayer open doors to glorify God and become testimonies to draw others to Him.

I share these stories not to brag or promote any form of prosperity gospel but to encourage you to see God moving in practical ways. I am convinced I would not be where I am today without the power, revelation, and application of prolonged consecrated fasting. I am also convinced that you will never be the same once you embark on fasting journeys of twenty-one to forty days. As God says in Jeremiah 29:13, "You will seek me and find me when you seek me with all your heart." Stay consistent, fast with a hunger for Jesus, and you, too, will see God's hand at work in your life.

Revival

And this gospel of the kingdom will be proclaimed
throughout the whole world as a testimony to all
nations, and then the end will come.
—Matthew 24:14

Finally, the results on your personal life of fasting will spark a revival in your family, friends, neighbors, strangers, cities, states, and the world. It started with you. You embarked on the journey of a pro-longed consecrated fast. God will honor your fast. Your changed life will be a witness to those around you. Jesus will give you the power to be a witness to others. When the opportunities arise and God opens the door, share your journey of fasting and encourage others to fast themselves or join you on the next prolonged consecrated fast.

Fasting clears the way in your heart to die to self, purify your heart, and find your calling, and now you can start leading others through these fasts and pray for the salvation of the lost in the world. In addition to that, fasting gives you the boldness to stop sitting around and start impacting the world for Jesus.

It will have a trickle effect on your family. People in your family will start encountering Jesus in supernatural ways or through your small acts of love. You become a vessel, contending for the faith of other people. You will begin to see moves of the Holy Spirit in your life, house, Bible studies, schools, sports teams, the government, churches, and the lost all across the world.

If you've been praying and fasting for someone to find Jesus, they will encounter Him. Remember, some fruits of the fast may not be seen until many years later. The journey of a forty-day fast is so powerful that it will purify your generational lines, your children's children, to the hundredth generation, and until the return of Jesus. You may not live long enough to see cities break out in revival, but rest assured your fasting has sparked a revival somewhere. It isn't about large gatherings or numbers or impacting a ton of people. Revival is change in your own life, impacting those around you.

> About a month into being born again, I decided to do my first-ever fast: a one-day fast with my spiritual mentor. At the start of the fast, my mentor asked me to pray and ask the Lord who He wanted me to pray for; multiple times, I heard in my heart my sister's name, Sarah. I

lengthened my fast to forty-eight hours and continued in constant prayer for my sister. Within three or four days of the fast ending, my sister, who was across the country, gave her life to Jesus and got baptized in the Holy Spirit.

—Colin Goebel

CHAPTER 10: MAINTAINING A FASTED STATE

Fasting draws you close to Jesus. It is a time to reset your life, receive spiritual, physical, emotional, and mental healing, break free from strongholds, remove idols, and transform your understanding of food. It shatters old habits and forms new habits on every level. It builds spiritual muscle memory. However, you must diligently maintain those habits beyond the fast in your daily life.

It is easy to fall back into old habits (especially with food) after breaking a fast. Therefore, maintaining a fasted state is crucial to receive the full benefits of fasting and continued spiritual growth.

This may not make much sense if you haven't completed a prolonged consecrated fast of twenty-one to forty days. The longer you fast, the greater you'll grow in discernment in flesh versus spirit. The stronghold of food and diet is highlighted because long fasts bring heightened spiritual sensitivity. That means letting the Holy Spirit guide you every day instead of following your own desires—learning to do what God wants, not what your flesh wants, and living according to His teachings.

"Humility, obedience, and spiritual hunger for God's Word and His ways are the common denominators of a fasted life that cultivates a lifestyle of intimacy and power with God."[41]

When you're in a fasted state, spiritually, you will be hungry for the things of God. You will sense the hunger of the Holy Spirit within you to pray, read the Bible, worship, die to yourself, love others, share the gospel, and have a deep, unquenched desire to be in God's presence all day. You and Jesus will be all that matters. The things you previously used to run to for comfort will no longer have a grip on your life. Keep it that way. If you prayed for twenty-one days straight during a fast, you might continue praying regularly afterward, even if it's just for a short time each day.

Physically, your body will feel brand new, invigorated, functionally proper, and full of energy. You won't need to eat three meals a day or a rich diet. Your body will desire living, healthy foods. When you don't feel hungry, don't mindlessly eat and snack; instead, pray. Your body is the temple of the Holy Spirit (1 Corinthians 6:19). It has been cleansed of toxins and impurities and is brand new. You have made space for the Holy Spirit to dwell freely and close inside of you.

It is far easier to maintain a fasted state if you maintain a healthy diet, stick to fruits and vegetables provided by the Lord, and avoid overeating or junk food. I also encourage you to maintain a vegan diet and stay away from meat. "Most Americans eat far too much meat—and over 95 percent of our exposure to dioxins comes from eating commercial animal fats."[42] I'm not saying our salvation in any way depends on what you eat, but I know from experience that indulging in unhealthy food can make you feel disconnected from God. Honor the Holy Spirit with your new temple (1 Corinthians 6:20). Treat it with the utmost care and watch the foods you put inside your body.

Mentally, you will be able to gather your thoughts. Any mental illness will be a thing of the past. You will be able to capture the lies of the enemy and cast them out. God will give you a sound mind (2 Timothy 1:7). You will be able to understand, think clearer, solve problems, communicate better, and focus. You will gain wisdom and grow in intelligence. You are a new wineskin now, and Jesus wants to continue to pour new wine into you.

Emotionally, you will have peace, contentment, and patience. You will be able to understand people's perspectives, and the fruits of the Holy Spirit will overflow from within your heart.

After a fast, there is usually a strong temptation to return to old unhealthy habits (strongholds of eating for comfort, overeating, eating junk food or rich diets). Remember: Food is one of the greatest human needs *and* one of the most subtle strongholds. It can become a stumbling block that causes you to fall back into the leading of your flesh and away from the leading of the Holy Spirit. Indulging in food for any other reason than the necessity to live opens the door to giving into your flesh. Temptations begin to creep back through old habits. This can potentially lead you back into sin, and that sin can destroy your life (James 1:14–17).

The tension over food often makes it harder to stay spiritually focused. That's why it's important to remember Romans 8:14–15, which says that as children of God, we are to be led by the Holy Spirit and should not fall back into fear or old ways. Instead, we should seek to do what pleases God.

Food is not evil. Eating is not a sin. God created people with physical appetites, and food is a gift. Food primarily should serve as a means to meet the nutritional needs of the body by providing strength and health. It is a time to celebrate God's goodness as well.

Maintaining a fasted state means not returning to your old life but continuing to grow spiritually and seek God's will. Sometimes you might need to fast again to regain spiritual sensitivity, especially if you start overindulging in your physical appetites or if you feel yourself being consumed by food and falling back into poor eating habits. The enemy may try to attack you with lies and confusion, steal joy and passion, or add unnecessary comforts to your life to distract you from growing closer to Jesus and cause you to fall back on relying on food for comfort.

You can still maintain a fasted state by staying spiritually sensitive to the Holy Spirit through daily prayer, reading the Bible, and worship, but when you feel your flesh taking over, go back to doing some daily shorter fasts.

One of the great evangelists, Charles Finney, fasted frequently and consistently. "He said that whenever he found the battery charge of the Spirit going down, when he felt the anointing of the Spirit weakening, he would go immediately into a three-day fast and that he would always end those fasts feeling recharged."[43]

Keep the fire burning by staying spiritually active. If you gained a deeper understanding of God's will and purpose for your life during your fast, share His message with others. You will feel fulfilled and motivated to keep going. And if you start to feel spiritually cold or lacking motivation to serve God, that may be a sign that it's time to return to fasting.

Surrendered to Christ

Remember all of the lessons you learned during your fast. Build some good habits in your life as you strive to continually grow spiritually. There's always room for more growth, always more to learn about God and His will. If you focus on that, you can prevent yourself from slipping back into old habits. In the limited time you have on this earth, each fasting journey you walk through will be unique, and you will discover more about yourself, more about Jesus, and get one step closer to Him.

As you maintain a fasted state, you'll learn to hear and follow the Lord's voice, and in turn, you will become more sensitive to His guidance in your daily life. Stay in His Word. Hebrews 4:12 says,

"The word of God is living and active, sharper than any two-edged sword, piercing to the division of soul and of spirit, of joints and of marrow, and discerning the thoughts and intentions of the heart." And Psalm 119:105 tells us, "Your word is a lamp for my feet, a light on my path." The Holy Spirit will continue to purify your heart and lead you on a path to continue to draw closer to Jesus.

Additionally, 1 Thessalonians 5:17 tells us to pray continually. Prayer is a conversation with Jesus, where we speak *and* listen, so be attentive to His guidance and promptings. Be quick to hear and slow to speak, as advised in James 1:19. That will help you discern God's voice amidst the noise of life. Jesus only acted and spoke what the Father told Him (John 5:19; 12:49). He didn't do more or less, and you are now at a place to do and say only what the Holy Spirit leads you to do.

God speaks to us in various ways, as noted in Job 33:14, so we need to remain sensitive to His leading. And Colossians 4:2 encourages us to devote ourselves to prayer, being watchful and thankful. That is how we stay in constant communion with Jesus.

Ultimately, as expressed in Galatians 2:20, maintaining a fasted state means living a life surrendered to Christ. As Paul writes, "I have been crucified with Christ. It is no longer I who live, but Christ who lives in me. And the life I now live in the flesh I live by faith in the Son of God, who loved me and gave himself for me." Our lives are no longer about our own desires but about living by faith and allowing Christ to guide our every step. These principles serve as a foundation for staying spiritually attuned and led by the Holy Spirit, whether we are fasting, breaking a fast, or in between fasts.

I'll leave you with this final story. It's easy to fall back into patterns of sin. This was the case for the Israelites. They were slaves in the land of Egypt for 430 years (Exodus 12:40) and were forced into brutal labor (Exodus 1:13–14). Think about working long daily shifts with little to no rest. No weekend breaks. No vacation. Little to no pay.

This was the situation for the Israelites until God delivered them from bondage.

They were now free in the wilderness. God provided them with food. However, they grew tired of this food and developed a strong craving for the foods they used to eat back in Egypt (Numbers 11:4–6). They complained. All they could think about was eating the rich foods they once had. They were even upset that God had freed them (Numbers 11:20), to the point they wished they were back in Egypt. The craving for food was so strong that it removed common sense. The people would have rather been back in bondage, getting beaten, working brutal labor, just so they could indulge in all the food they wanted.

Don't be like the Israelites God set free. The fast has renewed your life. Your body is new. You have received new wineskin. You are walking in freedom from bondage. Don't go back to old sins or eating habits. The rich diet of meats and processed junk will only bring you back to your old ways. Forsaking the results of the fast and returning to unhealthy eating and a sensual lifestyle is like forsaking God, complaining, and wanting to have nothing to do with Him, just so you can go back to indulging in food.

The stronghold of food will continue to be a battle, and it may take many fasting journeys before you break free. Romans 12:2 says, "Do not be conformed to this world, but be transformed by the renewal of your mind, that by testing you may discern what is the will of God, what is good and acceptable and perfect."

Not being conformed means not letting culture, politics, or social media (the world) guide you or tell you what to think about food. The world refers to time, the period of the age, the times you're living in, and the culture. Don't be molded by culture, the evil and ungodly spirits of the times. If you follow them, you lose your distinctiveness, uniqueness, and anointing, because if you become just like the times, people won't be able to see Jesus. You will lose your fragrance of love, become the odor of garbage of the world, and blend right in.

Let fasting renew your understanding of food. Test it out. It will take time to renew your mind about food and eating, but you will never be the same. Once you get free and experience God fully on every level—physically, spiritually, mentally, and emotionally—no craving or amount of food will ever be worth it.

> My first prolonged fast was forty-one days at the age of sixty-five. Before fasting for forty-one days, I prepared by fasting without food or water for three days. I took a day off, ate a little, and drank water. Then I started the forty-one-day fast. The first days, I had some minor headaches. I prayed multiple times daily, at home and at work. I felt the power of the Holy Spirit every time in my heart.
>
> Around day thirty-five, I started to feel hungry. I had a nightmare dream of seeing huge hamburgers. I took a bite and thought I broke the fast. From this point, I could not drink regular water. I started to drink distilled water, and that was good for me. I pressed through in prayer, which gave me the power to push through. I didn't feel hungry or thirsty and had the energy to work.
>
> At this time, I had an appointment to see my doctor for a checkup. I did all the blood and urine tests. They noticed I lost forty-nine pounds. I told them I was fasting, and I was on day thirty-eight with only water and no food. The doctor didn't want to believe me. He called in two nurses, and I shared my testimony. Everybody was surprised, but one nurse confirmed it was possible. She'd heard about fasting for ten to fifteen days, but forty-one days was a miracle.

When I finished forty-one days, I shared this testimony with brothers in churches. They started fasting. Some went on for seven days, and others told me I was going to die. I told them nobody can die from fasting. When I finished, I was stronger, more patient, and felt more power spiritually. I had positivity in my life and for my family.

The following year, I completed another forty-day fast. Since these prolonged fasts, I continue to do a minimum twenty-one-day fast every year. It has benefited me in growing in my faith and staying strong from attacks of Satan trying to destroy my faith.

—Vasile Trinca Sr.

CONCLUSION

My final message to you is a simple encouragement: You can do it. You can embark on a fasting journey, even as long as forty days. You might have to start with small steps, like skipping a meal or gradually reducing your eating habits to one meal a day. But you have the ability to do this.

It's important to shift your mindset away from what the culture or even the church might have taught you about fasting and understand its true biblical meaning. God calls all of us to surrender our lives to Him, not just acknowledging Him as our Savior but making Him the Lord of our lives.

Fasting can bring greater clarity and truth and help you understand God's love and purpose for you. Whether you've never considered giving your life to Jesus or you've felt distant from Him, fasting can ignite a new or renewed hunger and passion in your relationship with Him.

I've shared my own experiences to encourage you to take this first big step. Your journey may look different from mine, but I assure you it will change your life. Your perspective on eating, food, your body, relationships, and your connection with Jesus will never be the same once you commit to this path. Ultimately, fasting is a way to turn away from food for a period and to walk closer with Jesus, to encounter Him in a powerful way so that you can discern His will, trust Him, and follow Him.

Here are some additional fasting resources I recommend:
- *The Fasting Prayer* by Franklin Hall
- *Atomic Power with God thru Fasting and Prayer* by Franklin Hall
- *Fasting for Spiritual Breakthrough* by Elmer L. Towns
- *A Fasted Life* by Philip Renner
- *The Hidden Power of Prayer and Fasting* by Mahesh Chavda
- *The Miracle of Fasting* by Paul C. Bragg and Patricia Bragg
- *The Power of Prayer and Fasting* by Ronnie W. Floyd
- *A Complete Guide to Biblical Fasting* by Ted Shuttlesworth Jr.
- *God's Chosen Fast* by Arthur Wallace
- *Fasting and Eating for Health* by Joel Fuhrman
- *Rational Fasting* by Arnold Ehret
- *The Science and Fine Art of Fasting* by Herbert M. Shelton

These books offer a variety of perspectives on fasting, covering topics like spiritual breakthroughs, health benefits, and historical practices. If you want to learn more about the ancient practice, check them out.

ABOUT THE AUTHOR

Louis is of American Romanian descent, born and raised in Chicago, Illinois. He was a professional football player for the St. Louis and Los Angeles Rams. He had a radical encounter with Jesus in the Philippines in February 2020, where he fully surrendered his life to Jesus. He graduated with a master's in Christian studies from Dallas Theological Seminary. He is a full-time witness for Jesus. He travels all over the world to share the love of Jesus, preach the gospel, teach the Bible, equip and train churches, lead mission trips, disciple people, guide people through fasts, and help people grow in their relationship with Jesus.

ENDNOTES

Introduction
1. https://www.worldchristiandatabase.org.
2. John D. Barry, David Bomar, Derek R. Brown, and Rachel Klippenstein (eds), *Lexham Bible Dictionary* (Lexham Press, 2016).

Chapter 1
3. https://www.studylight.org/lexicons/eng/hebrew/6684.html.
4. https://biblehub.com/hebrew/6684.htm.
5. "The Place of Fasting in the Christian Life," C.S. Lewis Institute, accessed September 21, 2024, https://www.cslewisinstitute.org/resources/the-place-of-fasting-in-the-christian-life/.
6. "When You Fast, Part 3: Did Jesus Say Fasting Was Optional?" The Psalms Project Blog, accessed September 21, 2024, https://thepsalmsproject.com/blog/when-you-fast-part-3-did-jesus-say-fasting-was-optional.
7. Arthur Wallis, *God's Chosen Fast: A Spiritual and Practical Guide to Fasting* (CLC Publications, 2011), 21.
8. Jason Fung, MD, with Jimmy Moore, *The Complete Guide to Fasting: Heal Your Body Through Intermittent, Alternate-Day, and Extended Fasting* (Victory Belt Publishing, 2016), 53.

9. Don Colbert, MD, *Toxic Relief: Restore Health and Energy Through Fasting and Detoxification* (Siloam, 2012), 34–35.

10. Don Colbert, MD, *Toxic Relief: Restore Health and Energy Through Fasting and Detoxification* (Siloam, 2012), 38.

11. Scot McKnight, *Fasting*, Part 1: Spirituality and Fasting, 17.

12. Stephen R. Miller, *Daniel*, Vol. 18, The New American Commentary (Broadman & Holman Publishers, 1994).

13. The Holy Bible: English Standard Version (Crossway Bibles, 2016), Daniel 9:3.

14. Stephen R. Miller, *Daniel*, Vol. 18, The New American Commentary (Broadman & Holman Publishers, 1994), 278.

15. Mike Bickle with Dana Candler, *The Rewards of Fasting: Experiencing the Power and Affections of God* (Forerunner Publishing, 2013), 91.

16. Jason Fung, MD, with Jimmy Moore, *The Complete Guide to Fasting: Heal Your Body Through Intermittent, Alternate-Day, and Extended Fasting* (Victory Belt Publishing, 2016), 75.

17. Kevin Loria, Business Insider, "The True Story of a Man Who Survived Without Any Food for 382 Days," ScienceAlert, February 27, 2017, https://www.sciencealert.com/the-true-story-of-a-man-who-survived-without-any-food-for-382-days.

18. Oxford English Dictionary, "abstinence," accessed Thursday, January 30, 2025, https://www.oed.com/search/dictionary/?scope=Entries&q=abstinence&tl=true; F. L. Cross and Elizabeth A. Livingstone, eds., *The Oxford Dictionary of the Christian Church*, 3rd ed. (Oxford University Press, 2005), 8.

19. H. M. Shelton, *The Science and Fine Art of Fasting* (Mockingbird Press, 2019).

20. David M. Krasner, "Controlled Fasting Treatment for Schizophrenia," *Journal of Orthomolecular Medicine* 3, no. 4 (1974): 4–12, https://isom.ca/wp-content/uploads/2020/01/JOM_1974_03_4_12_Controlled_Fasting_Treatment_for_Schizophrenia.pdf.

21. Jason Fung, MD, with Jimmy Moore, *The Complete Guide to Fasting: Heal Your Body Through Intermittent, Alternate-Day, and Extended Fasting* (Victory Belt Publishing, 2016), 41.

22. Jack Hayford, "Fasting: The Feast That Frees," Jack Hayford Ministries, January 25, 2015, https://www.jackhayford.org/teaching/articles/fasting-the-feast-that-frees.

Chapter 2

23. Camilla Klein, "The Ultimate Guide to Biblical Fasting: How to Fast as a Christian and Unlock Spiritual Breakthrough," Christian Educators Academy, December 22, 2023, https://christianeducatorsacademy.com/the-ultimate-guide-to-biblical-fasting-how-to-fast-as-a-christian-and-unlock-spiritual-breakthrough/.

24. "When You Fast, Part 3," The Psalms Project, https://thepsalmsproject.com/blog/when-you-fast-part-3-did-jesus-say-fasting-was-optional.

Chapter 3

25. Examples of three-day fasts without food and water come from Esther 4:16 and Acts 9:9.

26. Nahum Sarna, *Exodus*, JPS Torah Commentary (JPS, 1991), 220.

27. Mahesh Chavda, *The Hidden Power of Prayer and Fasting: Releasing the Awesome Power of the Praying Church* (Destiny Image Publishers, Inc., 1998), 109.

28. D. W. T. Brattston, "Fasting in the Earliest Church," *Restoration Quarterly* 53, Issue 4 (2011), 236–37, https://christianfastingritual.weebly.com/uploads/4/0/6/1/40610219/fasting_in_the_earliest_church.pdf

29. Mahesh Chavda, *The Hidden Power of Prayer and Fasting: Releasing the Awesome Power of the Praying Church* (Destiny Image Publishers, Inc., 1998), 145.

30. Kirsopp Lake, ed. and trans., *The Apostolic Fathers with an English Translation*, vol. 1, LCL (Harvard University Press, 1959).

31. Arthur Wallis, *God's Chosen Fast: A Spiritual and Practical Guide to Fasting* (CLC Publications, 2011), 85.

32. Franklin P. Hall, *Glorified Fasting* (Martino Fine Books, 2017), 58.

33. Rachael Ajmera, "8 Health Benefits of Fasting, Backed by Science," Healthline, updated September 22, 2023, https://www.healthline.com/nutrition/fasting-benefits#brain-function.

Chapter 5

34. Arnold Ehret, *Rational Fasting* (BN Publishing, 2014), 42, https://books.apple.com/us/book/rational-fasting/id926680591.

35. Ehret, *Rational Fasting*, 68, https://books.apple.com/us/book/rational-fasting/id926680591.

Chapter 7

36. H. M. Shelton, *The Science and Fine Art of Fasting* (Mockingbird Press, 2019).

Chapter 8

37. Franklin P. Hall, *Glorified Fasting: The ABC of Fasting* (Martino Fine Books, 2017), 19–21.

38. Seth Bailin, "Notes from the Tanglewood Fasting Center: Q&A with Loren Lockman," 11, accessed September 12, 2024, https://www.sethbailin.com/uploads/1/0/1/9/101901806/tanglewood_-_notes_full.pdf.

Chapter 9

39. John D. Barry and Owen Strachan, eds., *Lexham Survey of Theology* (Lexham Press, 2018).

40. James A. Brooks, *Mark,* Vol. 23, The New American Commentary (Broadman & Holman Publishers, 1991), 65.

Chapter 10

41. Philip Renner, *A Fasted Life: Living a Lifestyle of Intimacy and Power with God* (Harrison House Publishers, 2021), Introduction, 8, e-book.

42. Don Colbert, MD, *Toxic Relief: Restore Health and Energy Through Fasting and Detoxification* (Siloam, 2012), 43.

43. Mahesh Chavda, *The Hidden Power of Prayer and Fasting: Releasing the Awesome Power of the Praying Church* (Destiny Image Publishers, Inc.), 145.